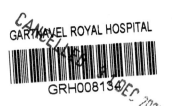

# Essential Philosophy of Psychiatry

Tim Thornton

Institute for Philosophy, Diversity and Mental Health,
University of Central Lancashire, UK

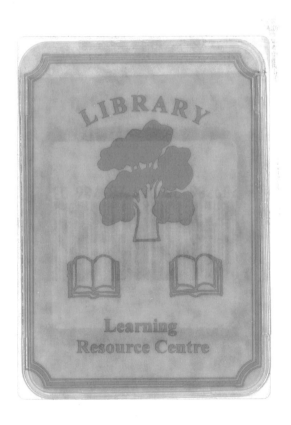

# OXFORD
UNIVERSITY PRESS

# OXFORD

UNIVERSITY PRESS

Great Clarendon Street, Oxford OX2 6DP

Oxford University Press is a department of the University of Oxford.
It furthers the University's objective of excellence in research, scholarship,
and education by publishing worldwide in

Oxford New York

Auckland Cape Town Dar es Salaam Hong Kong Karachi
Kuala Lumpur Madrid Melbourne Mexico City Nairobi
New Delhi Shanghai Taipei Toronto

With offices in

Argentina Austria Brazil Chile Czech Republic France Greece
Guatemala Hungary Italy Japan Poland Portugal Singapore
South Korea Switzerland Thailand Turkey Ukraine Vietnam

Oxford is a registered trade mark of Oxford University Press
in the UK and in certain other countries

Published in the United States
by Oxford University Press Inc., New York

© Oxford University Press 2007

The moral rights of the authors have been asserted

Database right Oxford University Press (maker)

First published 2007

British Library Cataloguing in Publication Data

Data available

Typeset by Cepha Imaging Private Ltd., Bangalore, India
Printed in Great Britain
on acid-free paper by
Ashford Colour Press Ltd, Gosport, Hampshire.

ISBN 978–0–19–922871–3

10 9 8 7 6 5 4 3 2

## Dedication

To my parents Mij and Grahame Thornton,
for everything.

# Foreword

I am delighted to welcome Tim Thornton's *Essential Philosophy of Psychiatry* as a most timely contribution to the rapidly expanding canon of the field. Tim's *Essentials*, as it will surely come to be called, is timely, first, just in being a short book. As such, it makes no claim to comprehensive coverage. In particular, like our more compendious *Oxford Textbook*, the focus of Tim's book is analytic rather than Continental philosophy. All the same, the very success of the new philosophy of psychiatry, developing as it is in so many and such diverse directions, practical as well as theoretical, demands some attempt at synthesis and overview. This is what Tim's book gives us. There is no dumbing down. Rather, key debates – about concepts of disorder, value theory and ethics, in the philosophy of science, and in the philosophy of mind – are presented with a remarkable economy and directness of style that allows those new to the discipline to gain a well-balanced understanding of the issues, while at the same time providing many fresh insights for established players.

Tim's *"Essentials"* is timely, too, in identifying and drawing out three closely related themes that are, indeed, essential to the new philosophy of psychiatry: the irreducible role of individual judgment, the importance of the whole person as the basic unit of meaning, and the need for an enriched conception of nature, a "relaxed naturalism" as Tim calls it, one in which personal meanings have as full a place as causal generalisations.

None of these three themes is incontestable, of course. To the contrary, a key role of philosophy in psychiatry is, precisely, to sustain an open and inclusive culture of debate, a dynamic of difference, firmly resistant to premature closure on this or that received authority. Correspondingly, the three themes that emerge from Tim's book, should be understood not as a settled 'corpus' for the new philosophy of psychiatry, but rather as a three-stranded golden thread running through the book as a whole. The golden thread is evident, for example, in the values-out *versus* values-in moves at the heart of the current debate about concepts of disorder, this being an aspect of the wider reductionism *versus* anti-reductionism debate in psychiatry; the thread appears again in the crucial shift from codified ethics to respect for individual values on which the clinical skills underpinning values-based practice are premised; it becomes fully explicit in the crucial roles of clinical judgement and of tacit knowledge alongside generalised research findings in a mature model of evidence-based practice; and it is of central importance at the interface between philosophy of mind and the new neurosciences, notably in the repeated struggles of psychiatry to work within the "space of reasons" (as Wilfrid Sellars has called it) without cutting itself off from the well tried and tested resources for medicine – explanatory, predictive and therapeutic – of the natural sciences, traditionally understood.

Tim concludes his book with a prediction, among others, of a collaborative research programme that will combine enactivism, from current analytic philosophy of mind, with phenomenology, from Continental philosophy. Such collaborations are at the heart of the inclusive nature of the new philosophy of psychiatry. As a formal discipline, analytic philosophy has its own distinctive contributions of generality and rigour to bring to the party. But it was after all phenomenology, not analytic philosophy, that maintained through much of the twentieth century a strong anti-reductionism, as now reflected in Tim's three key themes against the reductionism of the psychiatry of the day. Moreover, even taken together, analytic and Continental philosophy, on which the new philosophy of psychiatry has thus far been built, represent only 25% of the rich diversity of cultures worldwide. In reclaiming his three key themes for analytic philosophy, therefore, Tim's book lays the foundations for a future philosophy of psychiatry that is fully inclusive, not only of analytic and Continental philosophy, but also of the many other great traditions of thought and practice to be found around the world as a whole.

Let me then add a prediction of my own. I predict that Tim's *Essential Philosophy of Psychiatry*, in reclaiming the three interwoven themes, of judgement, of persons and of an enriched meaningful natural science, for analytic philosophy, will be seen to have taken us a key step towards the development of a philosophy of psychiatry that is genuinely international in scope, is fit for purpose as the defining discipline of twenty-first century mental health and social care.

KWM (Bill) Fulford
DPhil FRCP FRCPsych
Professor of Philosophy and Mental Health, University of Warwick
Co-Director of the Institute for Philosophy, Diversity and Mental Health
University of Central Lancashire
Honorary Consultant Psychiatrist, University of Oxford
Special Adviser for Values-Based Practice
Department of Health,UK; and Editor PPP

# Preface

This book is based on a number of papers and other short pieces that I have written on the philosophy of psychiatry over the last few years, but I have had the time to rethink and weave the threads together anew whilst in post as Professor of Philosophy and Mental Health at the new Institute for Philosophy, Diversity and Mental Health at Uclan, the University of Central Lancashire.

I am thus particularly grateful to Kamlesh Patel (Head of the Institute's parent Centre for Ethnicity and Health), Eileen Martin (Dean of the Faculty of Health) and Chris Heginbotham (Professor of Mental Health Policy and Management), who together established the Institute. It is a mark of some intellectual foresight to establish a new centre of excellence in the philosophy of mental health and I would wish to congratulate them even if I had not benefited directly myself.

A number of people have given me good advice on the manuscript: Natalie Banner, Matthew Broome, Rachel Cooper, Bill Fulford, Richard Gipps, Julian Hughes, Peter Lucas and Phil Thomas. However, I have also gained enormously from formal and informal discussion over the years with the people— philosophers and practitioners—who make up the community of philosophy of mental health both nationally in the UK and internationally. Many thanks. You will know who you are.

My thanks as ever to Lois, my partner, for editing and generally improving the first draft of this book, as well as more generally helping make such work possible (including sharing Brix, still the best cat in the world).

However, I want to express particular thanks to Bill Fulford, who has given me considerable support, well beyond the call of duty, over the last ten years and without whom I would not have been able to write this text. (That said, he is in no way to blame for my Wittgensteinian–McDowellian foibles.)

# Contents List

Part III **Facts**

# Introduction

This book aims to set out the essentials of the new philosophy of psychiatry in six chapters looking at three broad areas: the role of values in diagnosis and treatment; the nature and limits of understanding meaning; and the factual and scientific underpinnings of psychiatry. However, before outlining these three themes in a little more detail and then summarising the chapters, it is worth noting three general characteristics of this field that mark it out from other areas of philosophy.

First, as I will describe further below, philosophy in the broadly analytic or Anglo-American tradition has only recently embraced and, in turn, been embraced by psychiatry but over the last ten years there has been considerable research activity. Signs of new activity include the establishment of the journal *Philosophy, Psychiatry and Psychology* in 1994, co-edited in the US and UK. There is now an annual series of International Conferences on Philosophy, Psychiatry and Psychology, which have been held recently in Florence, Heidelberg, Yale and Leiden, and conferences are planned up to 2013. Another sign is the new series to which this book belongs, International Perspectives in Philosophy and Psychiatry, which also includes the recent and substantial *Oxford Textbook of Philosophy and Psychiatry*.

Secondly, however, philosophy of psychiatry is not a 'natural kind'. That is, there is not an established set of inter-related problems with familiar, if rival, solutions. Published work is instead generally drawn from parent sub-disciplines within philosophy, such as philosophy of mind, of science, and of values and ethics. It is an area of application, and also an area to test more abstract philosophical methods, accounts and theories. That means, however, that I have had to make real choices as to what to include in this book and the selection, inevitably, reflects some personal interests that would not be shared by all researchers in the field.

Thirdly, unlike some areas of philosophy, philosophy of psychiatry can have a real impact on practice. It is a philosophy of and for mental health care. It provides tools for critical understanding of contemporary practices, of the assumptions on which mental health care more broadly, and psychiatry more narrowly, are based. It is an area where philosophical work is carried out by practitioners and service users, as well as professional philosophers.

These features mark the subject out as one in flux, responding to changes in the broader social and political context of mental health care, as well as to developments in other areas of philosophy. At the end of the book I will speculate about future developments in philosophy of psychiatry.

Although my aim in this book is to introduce the philosophy of psychiatry and to provide an overview of some of the key debates, I have not attempted to be neutral. Whilst I aim to set out the attractions of and motivations for adopting the various competing views summarised throughout this book, my own overall views will be apparent. I make no apology for this. Philosophy of psychiatry is a contested discipline, and readers should expect to have to think through how they agree and disagree with the arguments set out in the books and research papers that make up the field. Although it provides an introductory survey, this book should be no exception to that need for a critical response from readers.

## Overview of the themes of the book: values, meanings and facts in psychiatry

As I have said, the new philosophy of psychiatry is a developing field within Anglo-American, broadly analytic philosophy. Whilst the father of psychopathology, the German psychiatrist and philosopher Karl Jaspers, combined psychiatric and philosophical expertise, within the English speaking tradition, philosophy and psychiatry went their separate ways throughout most of the twentieth century. (By contrast, in mainland Europe the connection between psychiatry and phenomenological philosophy has continued since Jaspers' day.)

However, towards the end of the twentieth century, the rise of the anti-psychiatry movement prompted a resurgence of analytic philosophical interest in psychiatry. This was because a key element of anti-psychiatric criticism of mental health care turned on a contentious claim about the nature of mental illness—that mental illness does not exist and is a myth. Such a sceptical claim is paradigmatically philosophical and one of the main proponents of anti-psychiatry, the psychiatrist Thomas Szasz, put forward a number of explicitly philosophical arguments in support of it.

His main argument turns on the claim that mental illness is defined by reference to evaluative norms by contrast with physical illness, which is defined as deviation from structural or functional integrity. Thus, he argued, it was logically absurd to think that mental illness could, like physical illness, be treated by medical means. Szasz' claims spurred responses by both psychiatrists and philosophers putting forward analyses of mental illness to undercut the sceptical argument. Thus, the analysis of mental illness and the question of whether it is essentially value-laden lie at the heart of recent philosophy of psychiatry.

That is not the only subject matter that calls for philosophical analysis, however nor even the only area where values play a key role. Mental health care is the only area of medicine where fully conscious adult patients of normal intelligence can be treated against their will. Especially against a general increase in the emphasis on the rights and voices of patients or service users (or subjects), this aspect of mental health care calls for justification. Just what is it, if anything, about mental illness that can sometimes justify such coercive treatment? Given also that the values in play in mental health care seem to be more divergent than in other areas of physical medicine, how are value judgements best understood?

A key theme in this book is therefore the role of *values* in psychiatry, both in the analysis of mental illness and, thus, in diagnosis, but also in the ethical justification for treatment and management in mental health care. In addition to values, however, there are two other important general themes in this book. Psychiatry has, since Jaspers' work, sought to balance two key elements: investigation of the bio-medical facts and investigation of subjects' experiences, and thus the two further broad themes of this book are *facts* and *meanings*.

Alongside bio-medical facts, meanings, broadly construed to include the nature of subjects' experiences, beliefs and utterances have somehow to be integrated into mental health care. This raises two general questions. First, what is the nature of understanding and what limits are placed on it within psychiatry? I examine this question in chapter 3, where I look at Jaspers' views on what he calls 'static' and 'genetic' understanding or empathy, and also more recent attempts to go beyond the limits placed on these by Jaspers. Secondly, how in general does meaning or content fit into a broader conception of nature? Chapter 4 examines and criticises two rival views relevant to mental health care: cognitivism within psychiatry and discursive psychology.

No account of the recent philosophy of psychiatry would be complete without some attention to two debates that have arisen from within psychiatric practice, which concern the scientific status of psychiatric facts. One is the concern with the status of psychiatric classification or taxonomy that has preoccupied the profession during the second half of the twentieth century, but which received further impetus in response to anti-psychiatry. The other concerns the more recent rise in evidence-based medicine in medicine in general, but also within mental health care.

Dividing the philosophy of psychiatry into values, meanings and facts is, to some extent, artificial. But it provides a basic framework to think about the range of subjects currently under discussion.

## Chapter outline

### Part I: Values

### 1. Anti-psychiatry, values and the philosophy of psychiatry

What role do values play in psychiatric diagnosis? This chapter outlines the recent revival of the philosophy of psychiatry as a response to Szsaz' criticisms of the very idea of mental illness as a myth. It examines Szasz' arguments based on the idea that mental and physical illness answer to distinct norms. Whilst physical illness is deviation from structural or functional integrity, mental illness, Szasz argues, depends on deviation from evaluative norms and thus mental illness cannot be treated by medical means. This view is contrasted with biologically-minded defences of psychiatry offered by Kendell and Boorse.

The second section sets out Fulford's diagnosis of the underlying agreement and disagreement between value-theorists like Szasz and descriptivists like Boorse and Kendell. Both sides implicitly agree that physical illness is value-free, but Fulford argues that that assumption is mistaken. This leads him to a view of mental illness as akin to physical illness in being value-laden, but no less real for that. Fulford himself comes under fire from Pickering who argues that he subscribes to a 'likeness argument' that cannot, in fact, settle the status of mental illness. I argue, however, that Pickering construes the likeness argument in a foundational manner and that this can itself be rejected.

The third section examines Wakefield's harmful dysfunction analysis of disorder. This turns on analysing disorder in terms of dysfunction and explaining it in descriptive terms, as others have sought to do via evolutionary theory. Biological functions look to be a promising way of 'naturalising' the idea of mental disorder because they are both normative (there is a prescriptive distinction between behaviour that accords with them and that which does not), but also rooted in scientific theory. I argue, however, that the very idea of biological function presupposes, rather than explains normativity and thus fails to explain disorder in more basic terms.

The final section takes mild cognitive impairment as an example. The same general issues that concern mental illness as a whole apply to this difficult borderline condition, helping to underlie the real difficulty of making a judgement as to its pathological status.

## 2. Values, psychiatric ethics and clinical judgement

What underpins value and ethical judgements in psychiatry? This chapter begins by outlining the conventional tools deployed in medical ethics in general: principles-based accounts of ethical judgement in the form of deontology, consequentialism and the Four Principles approach. It then examines two key additional complexities found in psychiatry: the justification of compulsory treatment and the diversity of values found in practice. It outlines one proposal to explain how a key aspect of severe mental illness, at least, might be of the right kind to justify involuntary treatment. The section closes with a sketch of the key claims that underpin values-based practice: an approach to values diversity that is of growing influence in the UK and internationally.

The second section examines the model of values implicit in values-based practice. One possible explanation of differences of opinion in value judgements is that values are subjective, but I argue that it is better to think of value judgements as genuinely objective, which is, nevertheless, not codifiable in principles. That is, one should be particularist, rather than principlist, about values.

The third section compares this view of values-based practice with one of the most influential form of medical ethics in clinical practice: the Four Principles approach. Particularism about ethical judgements is further justified by questioning what it is that disciplines, as well as guides, ethical judgements. The resulting picture is one which places a central focus on having good judgement in the face of complex ethical situations, but where such judgement cannot be reduced to the algorithmic application of any principle.

## Part II: Meanings

### 3. Understanding psychopathology

What is the role and nature of understanding, by contrast with explanation, in psychiatry and does it have limits? The chapter starts with the historical origins of philosophy of psychiatry in Jaspers' philosophically charged account of understanding or empathy, which he divides into two kinds. *Static understanding* is the application of phenomenology to psychiatry to grasp the nature of psychological states: what they are like. *Genetic understanding* is the grasp of how one state can give rise to another in an ideally typical fashion that is shared empathically. Light can be shed on Jaspers' views of empathy by comparing them with a contemporary debate between 'theory theory' and 'simulation theory' in philosophy of mind.

Although he argues that empathy lies at the heart of psychiatry, Jaspers also thinks that there are principled limits on its application. It cannot be used to understand the content of what he calls 'primary' delusions, as these are stubbornly 'un-understandable'.

The second and longer section of the chapter examines a number of contemporary attempts in philosophy of psychiatry to resist Jaspers' professional pessimism and to articulate a route to understand the content of delusions on the basis of a number of rival philosophical models. I examine 5 models and conclude that, whilst they promise to shed some light on the phenomena, none offers a direct route to empathic understanding.

### 4. Theorising about meaning for mental health care

How can we explain the place of meaning—or the content of mental states—in nature? What kind of theoretical framework can shed light on meaning in mental health care? This chapter begins by contrasting two influential approaches.

The first section examines cognitivist accounts of meaning within psychiatry. According to these approaches, the meaning or content of mental states is carried by inner mental representations, which are processed by internal information processing systems within the brain. As an approach, it borrows from the rise of computer science and looks to be a scientifically respectable way of explaining the place of meaning in nature. This approach, however, faces a key challenge, which is to explain how inner states in the head can be about anything.

The second section of the chapter looks at a fundamentally different approach: a social constructionist form of discursive psychology. According to this approach, meaning is constructed primarily in utterances. It is constituted by public phenomena, rather than, as for cognitivism, by factors within the skull. Although constructionism about meaning is often justified by appeal to the work of the philosopher Ludwig Wittgenstein, I argue that, properly understood, his work provides both tools for criticising the substantial claims of constructionist discursive psychology and for showing why they are unnecessary.

The third section outlines a positive view of meaning and mental content derived from Wittgenstein. According to this view, meaning is an irreducible phenomenon, although grounded in practical abilities and shared judgements. This view is then contrasted with an alternative account of the significance of Wittgenstein for theorising about mental health recently put forward by Derek Bolton and Jonathan Hill.

## Part III: Facts

### 5. The validity of psychiatric classification

Is psychiatric classification valid? Starting with Hempel's seminal advice to the APA, the chapter looks at the relation of reliability and validity, and the connection to the debate about values in psychiatry from Chapter 1. It argues that only on the adoption of a specific philosophical model of values would the presence of values in psychiatric taxonomy undermine its validity.

The second section raises two particular challenges to psychiatric validity. The first is a criticism by Kendell and Jablensky based on the need for clear boundaries between syndromes. The second is the WPA's call for narrative formulations in comprehensive diagnosis.

The third section draws lessons from recent philosophy of science to place the debate about validity in context. It concludes with the suggestion that there are no external standards by which to assess psychiatric validity. There is no alternative to local judgement about the current state of the productive relation between psychiatric classification and theory. In the case of narrative formulations, the standard of validity is the standing obligation to reflect on the general concepts used to frame even person-specific narratives.

## 6. The relation of evidence-based medicine and tacit knowledge in clinical judgement

What is the status of evidence-based medicine in psychiatry? This chapter considers the status of EBM, exemplified in the hierarchy of forms of evidence, and considers the role of uncodified judgement alongside algorithmic rules.

Because EBM concerns how best to learn from experience, the chapter begins by looking at David Hume's challenge to justify induction. Hume's challenge is both disconcertingly simple and, for that very reason, disorientating. It appears to show that basing predictions for the future on past experience has no justification.

The second section looks at Hume's own brief positive account and contrasts it with John Stuart Mill's methods of eliminative induction. Mill's methods help shed light on the justification for randomised control trials and their effectiveness can be determined *a priori*. Thus, they promise to justify EBM's evidence hierarchy. Nevertheless, closer consideration reveals that the methods cannot be applied in practice and applying approximations of them requires prior epistemic judgements.

The final section looks in more detail at how judgements can be codified. It uses Wittgenstein's discussion of rule following to shed light on the ultimately practical grounding of even deductive judgements. However, this also shows how Hume's scepticism can be defused. This leaves EBM intact, and at the same time dependent not just on what can be codified in algorithmic methods, but also shared uncodified practical judgements.

# Part I

# **Values**

Chapter 1

# Anti-psychiatry, values and the philosophy of psychiatry

## Plan of the chapter

1. **The debate between 'values in' and 'values out' accounts of mental illness**
   Szasz' critique of mental illness as bodily illness
   Szasz' critique of the claim that mental illness is *sui generis*
   Kendell's and Boorse's 'values out' reactions

2. **Putting the debate into context**
   Fulford's overview of the role of values in psychiatry
   The status of the likeness argument

3. **A biological teleological model of mental illness**
   A teleological account of function?
   So can biological function be reduced?

4. **Mild cognitive impairment: a case study in philosophy of psychiatry**

5. **Conclusions**

Whilst, in mainland Europe, philosophy carried out in the phenomenological tradition retained a close connection to psychiatry throughout the 20th century, Anglo-American or broadly analytic philosophy largely lost touch. Analytic philosophy of psychiatry has been reborn in large part as a response to the rise of the anti-psychiatry movement in the 1960s. This was because, whatever its broader *political* underpinnings, the disagreement between anti-psychiatry and biologically-minded defences of psychiatry was a *philosophical*, rather than an empirical disagreement. It thus prompted a fresh philosophical examination of the nature and conceptual underpinnings of psychiatry.

At the heart of the debate about anti-psychiatry is a debate about the nature of mental illness itself. The anti-psychiatry view that mental illness does not exist has immediate repercussions for the justification of mental health care practice. Thus, the analysis of mental illness is not merely one question of interest to the philosophy of psychiatry, it is the key question. For that reason it is where I will begin.

The first section of the chapter examines Szasz' arguments based on the idea that mental and physical illness answer to distinct norms. Whilst physical illness is deviation from structural or functional integrity, mental illness, Szasz argues, depends on deviation from evaluative norms and thus mental illness cannot be treated by medical means. This view is contrasted with biologically-minded defences of psychiatry offered by Kendell and Boorse.

The second section describes two attempted overviews of the debate about mental illness. Fulford suggests that whilst value-theorists like Szasz, and descriptivists like Boorse and Kendell disagree about the status of mental illness they implicitly agree that physical illness is value-free. Fulford argues, however, that assumption is mistaken. He argues, instead, that illness as a whole is essentially value-laden, but mental illness appears more so because the values involved are more contested. Just because mental illness is value-laden, it does not follow that it is unreal.

Fulford himself comes under fire from Pickering who argues that he subscribes to a 'likeness argument', which cannot, in fact, settle the status of mental illness. I argue, however, that it is only because Pickering construes the likeness argument as foundationalist that his criticism of it seems to work, but supporters of the likeness argument need not assume that its premises are theory-free observations or data. It can still play a role even within a broadly holistic view of reasoning.

The third section examines Wakefield's harmful dysfunction analysis of illness. This turns on reducing mental disorder to a biological dysfunction itself analysed into the purely descriptive terms of evolutionary theory. Biological functions look to be a promising way of 'naturalising' the idea of mental disorder because they are both normative (there is a prescriptive distinction between behaviour that accords with them and that which does not), but also rooted in scientific theory. I argue, however, that the very idea of biological function presupposes the kind of intelligibility exemplified in reason-giving. It does not explain it. Thus, it fails to explain disorder in more basic terms.

The final section takes mild cognitive impairment as an example. The same general issues that concern mental illness as a whole apply to this difficult borderline condition helping to demonstrate the real difficulty of making a judgement as to its pathological status.

The debate about the nature of mental illness outlined in this chapter can usefully be characterised in two ways. On the one hand, a key disagreement between the protagonists is whether mental illness in particular, or illness more generally, is essentially evaluative. Does the analysis of mental illness contain reference to values or not? Some philosophers and psychiatrists (to whom I will refer as 'values in theorists' or 'value theorists' for short) argue that at the heart of the idea of illness is something that is either bad for a sufferer, or is a deviation from a social or moral norm. Both of these are evaluative notions and, hence, both are 'values in' views.

Others (descriptivists or 'values out' theorists) argue that it is what I will call a plainly factual matter. (I will use the word 'plain' to refer to a non-normative or austerely descriptive account.) Typically, they argue that illness involves a failure of a biological function and function—and hence deviation from, or failure of, function—is a plainly factual, biological term couched in evolutionary theory. Of course, disagreement about the presence or absence of values in the analysis is just one aspect of the debate. A further question is, for example, what follows from this for the objectivity of mental illness and the status of psychiatry as a science (Chapter 5 considers the implications of values for psychiatric validity).

A second useful characterisation links the debate about mental illness to other debates in philosophy about the place in nature of problematic concepts. On this second construal, the question is whether mental illness can be *naturalised*. That is, can mental illness be accommodated within a satisfactory conception of the natural realm?

The most common form of philosophical naturalism is reductionism, which attempts to show the place in our conception of nature of puzzling concepts by explaining them in terms of, and so reducing them to, basic concepts that are unproblematically natural. So on this second characterisation of the debate, a pressing question is whether, or to what extent, the concept of mental illness can be reduced to plainly factual concepts. If it cannot be naturalised, to what extent is it consistent with a scientific account of the world?

What makes reductionism difficult is that different concepts can seem to behave quite differently from one another. Take, for example, a distinction drawn from the work of the philosopher Wilfrid Sellars, and repopularised by John McDowell (McDowell 1994), between the 'realm of law' and the 'space of reasons'. Whilst the space of reasons concerns meaning-laden and normative phenomena that we take for granted in understanding minds, the realm of law concerns events that can be explained by subsuming them under natural scientific laws. In the philosophy of mind, reductionists attempt to show how the space of reasons can be completely explained using the resources of the realm of law. Anti-reductionists argue that the normativity of mental states and meanings—the fact that beliefs can rationalise and support one another, can be right or wrong—cannot be captured in terms, for example, of statistical laws of association.

In fact, value theorists in the debate about mental illness are making a similar point to anti-reductionists in the philosophy of mind. They argue that the very idea of mental illness is a normative notion—since values are normative and have a good versus bad dimension—and for that reason cannot be reduced to plainly factual or realm of law terms. I will characterise the recent debate about the status of mental illness using both the idea of it concerning 'values in versus values out' and the question of how to naturalise mental illness.

## 1. The debate between 'values in' and 'values out' accounts of mental illness

I will begin by outlining the US psychiatrist Thomas Szasz' critique of psychiatry. Although best known in psychiatric circles, Szasz' critique is not the only source of anti-psychiatric ideas. Both the historical analysis of Michel Foucault, which suggested continuity between historical forms of social control and contemporary psychiatric practice, and also the radical ideas about therapy of the British psychiatrist R. D. Laing, contributed to a debate starting in the 1960s and continuing to the present day about the status and legitimacy of psychiatry. However, Szasz' justification for the claim that mental illness itself is a myth has the most explicit philosophical argument.

The centrepiece of Szasz' critique is an article and then a book (containing the article) called *The Myth of Mental Illness*. Szasz claims that the everyday assumption that mental illnesses exist as much as physical illnesses do has two lines of support, both of which he rejects. One is based on the relation between mental illnesses and illnesses (or diseases) of the brain. The other depends on the idea of *sui generis* mental illnesses.

### Szasz' critique of the defence of mental illness as bodily illness

The first line of argument for the existence of mental illness is based on the reality of illnesses of the body or brain. It is drawn from the idea that, for example, 'syphilis of the brain' or 'delirious conditions' produce disorders of thinking and behaviour. The argument in defence of mental illness can now run as follows. If all mental illnesses are illnesses of the brain and if illnesses of the brain are real, then mental illnesses are real.

Szasz offers two criticisms of this argument. The first is that there is a distinction between the ability of neurological defects to explain bodily symptoms—a neurological defect might, for example, explain defects of vision—and their supposed ability to explain (normal or) abnormal thought: 'Explanations of this sort of occurrence—assuming that one is interested in the belief itself and does not regard it simply as a symptom or expression of something else that is more interesting—must be sought along different lines' (Szasz 1972: 13).

The second criticism is also based on drawing a distinction in this case between physical symptoms, such as fever or pain (sic) and mental symptoms. The latter, unlike the former, turn crucially on aspects of the relation between sufferer and clinician. If a subject reports that he or she is Napoleon, this only counts as a mental symptom if he or she is not Napoleon. This, in turn, Szasz suggests, involves a 'covert comparison between the patient's ideas ... and those of the observer and the society in which they live' (Szasz 1972: 14). It is worth noting that Szasz' argument goes a little too quickly in that it blurs the distinction between how we might *know* that a subject is deluded—perhaps by comparison with what we think—and what it *is* to be deluded. That is, he blurs epistemology and ontology here. The underlying point, however, is that assessment of mental symptoms is normative in a way that assessment of physical symptoms is not: 'The notion of mental symptom is therefore inextricably tied to the social, and particularly the ethical, context in which it is made, just as the notion of bodily symptom is tied to an anatomical context' (Szasz 1972: 14).

Taken together, these two criticisms are designed to head off the idea that mental illness can be defended by its relation to bodily illness:

> For those who regard mental symptoms as signs of brain disease, the concept of mental illness is unnecessary and misleading. If they mean that people so labelled suffer from diseases of the brain, it would seem better, for the sake of clarity, to say that and not something else (Szasz 1972: 14).

## Szasz' critique of the claim that mental illness is *sui generis*

What then of the idea that mental illness is *sui generis*: a form of illness like physical or bodily illness, but essentially and distinctly mental? Szasz offers two arguments, which I will here refer to as the swift argument and the longer argument. In fact, the swift argument can be interpreted in two ways.

Szasz suggests that the root of the claim that mental illness is *sui generis* is to think of mental illness as a 'deformity of the personality', which explains human disharmony or more generally life problems. His response to this idea is swift:

> Clearly, this is faulty reasoning, for it makes the abstraction 'mental illness' into a cause of, even though this abstraction was originally created to serve only as a shorthand expression for, certain types of human behaviour. (Szasz 1972: 15)

This swift argument depends on a premise that might very well be doubted: that putative mental illness is just the very same thing as a form of behaviour. This would be a form of behaviourism or, more specifically, mental illness behaviourism. If mental illness just is behaviour—a behaviourist claim—and if it is also supposed to cause that same behaviour then, because nothing can cause itself, there is a contradiction.

There is, however, a weaker and, thus, more plausible version of the swift argument, which starts from the assumption that there is merely a definitional connection between ascriptions of mental illness and relevant behaviour. This is still a kind of mental illness behaviourism, although weaker, and like logical behaviourism in the philosophy of mind might be taken to preclude a causal connection between mental illness and behaviour. Why?

Since the seminal analysis of causation provided by the Scottish philosopher David Hume it has been widely held that causal connections are contingent connections: they do not hold of necessity. Thus, to take an example from Hume, whilst bread nourishes—a causal relation: it causes the body to be nourished—it *might not* have done so. Such contingency is an essential feature of causation. Thus, if the connection between a putative cause and its effect is not contingent, but necessary, then it cannot be genuinely causal.

The argument in the case of mental illness can now be stated as follows. If mental illness is defined in terms of certain sorts of behaviour then the connection between it and those forms of behaviour is necessary not contingent. Thus, it cannot cause that behaviour, but that is what it was supposed to do. Thus, there is no such thing. I will return to this second version of the swift argument shortly having introduced the longer argument.

The second related, but longer argument that Szasz deploys against a *sui generis* conception of mental illness runs as follows:

> The concept of illness, whether bodily or mental, implies deviation from some clearly defined norm. In the case of physical illness, the norm is the structural and functional integrity of the human body. Thus, although the desirability of physical health, as such, is an ethical value, what health is can be stated in anatomical and physiological terms. What is the norm, deviation from which is regarded as mental illness? This question cannot be easily answered. But whatever this norm may be, we can be certain of only one thing: namely, that it must be stated in terms of psychological, ethical, and legal concepts ... [W]hen one speaks of mental illness, the norm from which deviation is measured is a *psychosocial and ethical* standard. Yet the remedy is sought in terms of *medical* measures that—it is hoped and assumed—are free from wide differences of ethical value. The definition of the disorder and the terms in which its remedy are sought are therefore at serious odds with one another ... (Szasz 1972: 15)

> Since medical interventions are designed to remedy only medical problems, it is logically absurd to expect that they will help solve problems whose very existence have been defined and established on non-medical grounds (Szasz 1972: 17).

Thus, there are two separate and incompatible sets of norms, deviation from which supposedly constitutes illness. On the one hand, there are structural and functional norms for physical or bodily illness. On the other hand, there are psychological, psychosocial, ethical and legal norms for supposed mental illnesses. The problem, according to Szasz, is that subscribers to the idea of mental illness also insist that it can be addressed using medical measures, but these are designed for, or perhaps characterised by reference to, the structural and functional norms of bodily illness. That is why it is 'logically absurd' to expect them to be appropriate. It is a kind of 'category error' (in the phrase of the philosopher Gilbert Ryle 1949).

There would be no difficulty if subscribers to the idea of mental illness did not also insist that it can be addressed using medical measures. Szasz himself does not deny the existence of the phenomena that are taken to constitute mental illness in this sense. They are real life problems:

> While I maintain that mental illnesses do not exist, I obviously do not imply or mean that the social and psychological occurrences to which the label is attached also do not exist. Like the personal and social troubles that people had in the Middle Ages, contemporary human problems are real enough. It is the labels we give them that concern me, and, having labelled them, what we do about them (Szasz 1972: 21).

Szasz' second argument has two stages either of which might be criticised. One might dispute the idea that mental illness turns on a different kind of norm to physical illness. Later in this chapter, I will outline Wakefield's recent model of mental disorder as based on a failure of biological function of some sort. Such an account, if successful, would help to block Szasz' first premiss. For now, I wish instead to suggest that there is a way to address the second step of the argument: that, on the assumption that mental illnesses are constituted by deviation from distinct psycho-social or ethical norms, it is logically absurd to treat them using 'medical' means, and thus the idea that there are illnesses so constituted and so treatable is false or a myth.

It is helpful, to begin with, to think again of the swift argument against mental illness outlined earlier. Szasz claims that mental illnesses are defined by reference to behaviour because they are used to identify features of, or more specifically deformities of, personality. However, they are also invoked *causally* to explain those disturbances, but either:

- since nothing can cause itself, such a construal of mental illness is inconsistent; or
- since causal connections are contingent, but definitional connections are necessary then mental illness cannot cause abnormal behaviour and, again, such a construal of mental illness is inconsistent.

From this it would also follow that there is nothing that a medical intervention can be brought into causal contact with.

Clearly, the strength of either version of this swift argument depends on the premiss that mental illnesses really are merely shorthand for behaviour—a kind of mental illness behaviourism. The main support for the premiss appears to be that mental illness is diagnosed via behaviour. But that is consistent with a position that is more plausible than mental illness behaviourism. This is to say that, although mental illnesses are identified through behaviour, they are not identical to that behaviour, but are instead its underlying cause.

In the philosophy of mind—where behaviourism proper was much discussed in the 1960s—the American philosopher Donald Davidson (1917–2003) defended, against behaviourism, a conception of mental states in general of just this alternative sort. As he points out, we often describe events by their effects. The act of firing a gun may also be described as an act of murdering a president. The same is true of describing mental states. We may describe them in terms of behaviour. This does not require, however, a behaviourist identification of mental states and behaviour. Mental states might be picked out by their effects—such as actions—whilst still being distinct from, and even the causes of, them.

Against the claim that causal connections are contingent, whereas definitional connections express necessities, Davidson points out a fundamental distinction. Necessary connections depend on how they are described. Causal connections depend on the fabric of the world. Thus, if firing the gun causes the death of the president then we can label the event of firing the gun 'the cause of the death of the president'. We can report the causal connection by saying 'firing the gun caused the death of the president' or equally by swapping 'firing the gun' and 'the cause of the death of the president' we can report the same events: 'the cause of the death of the president caused the death of the president'.

This second claim is, however, a necessary truth. It is necessarily true that the cause of the death of the president caused the death of the president, but that fact does not undermine the contingent causal connection expressed in the first claim. It does not block the idea that a real event caused his death.

In the case of mental illnesses, one might object against Szasz that although mental illnesses are identified through behaviour they are not identical to that behaviour. Thus, there is no intrinsic difficulty with the idea of mental illnesses causing abnormal behaviour. This disarms both versions of the swift argument. It also suggests a way to respond to the second longer argument.

The response runs as follows. Although mental illnesses are identified through behaviour (including linguistic behaviour) they are not identical to that behaviour. Thus, although the norms that play an essential role in the identification of mental illnesses may be distinct from those that identify physical illnesses—they are psychosocial, ethical and legal, rather than structural and functional—that identifying role does not preclude a causal role for mental illness. Thus, it is not logically absurd to expect medical treatment of mental illness and, thus, the model of mental illness that combines these two features—identification according to psychosocial norms and medical treatability—is not absurd and has not been shown to be false or mythical.

These responses to both of Szasz' arguments identified above undermine his conclusion that mental illness is unreal and a myth, but they do not undermine the key claim that mental illness is constituted by essentially evaluative norms. (It is also worth noting that Szasz himself has recently claimed that the proposition that mental illness is a myth was not a conclusion to an argument he offered but something he accepted as a premiss (2004: 321).)

If it is true that mental illness is essentially evaluative then that claim might seem to underwrite other substantial claims about the nature of psychiatry. Perhaps, for example, it serves to show that psychiatry cannot aspire to scientific status, on the assumption either that the methods of science are value-free or that science concerns objective features of the world whilst values are subjective. These further connections will be discussed in Chapter 5. I will now outline two opponents to Szasz' starting point who offer instead descriptivist value-free analyses of illness.

## Kendell's and Boorse's 'values out' reactions

Two influential defences of the idea of mental illness were offered in 1975 by the Christopher Boorse and Robert Kendell. Like Thomas Szasz, R. E. Kendell was a Professor of Psychiatry, but unlike Szasz, Kendell was an establishment figure. After his time as Professor of Psychiatry at Edinburgh University, he became Chief Medical Officer for Scotland and was elected President of the Royal College of Psychiatrists in the UK.

In a paper called 'The concept of disease and its implications for psychiatry', he argues in defence of mental illnesses or diseases by suggesting a method for assessing the status of mental illness:

> before we can begin to decide whether mental illnesses are legitimately so called we have first to agree on an adequate definition of illness; to decide if you like what is the defining characteristic or the hallmark of disease. (Kendell 1975a: 306)

Reviewing the history of the debate he comments:

> By 1960 the 'lesion' concept of disease, and its associated assumptions of a single cause and a qualitative difference between sickness and health had been discredited beyond redemption, but nothing had yet been put in its place. It was clear, though, that its successor would have to be based on a statistical model. (Kendell 1975a: 309)

As Kendell goes on to say, whilst a statistical model may address some of the weaknesses of a single lesion model, statistical abnormality by itself cannot distinguish between 'deviations from the norm which are harmful, like hypertension, those which are neutral, like great height, and those which are positively beneficial, like superior intelligence' (Kendell 1975a: 309). Some further criterion is needed to address the fact that illness is a specific kind of deviation from the norm.

Kendell's preferred solution, in this paper, is based on the work of the British chest physician, J. G. Scadding:

> Scadding was the first to recognise the need for a criterion distinguishing between disease and other deviations from the norm that were not matters for medical concern, and suggested that the crucial issue was whether or not the abnormality placed the individual at a 'biological disadvantage'. Although he was primarily concerned with defining individual diseases, his definition of *a* disease has clear implications for the global concept. He defines illness not by its antecedents—the aetiological agent or the lesion producing the overt manifestations—but by its consequences. In itself this is not new; previous attempts to define illness as a condition producing suffering or as meriting medical intervention had done the same but... [had] proved inadequate. The concept of 'biological disadvantage' differs from these, however, in being more fundamental and less obviously an epiphenomenon, and in being immune to the idiosyncratic personal judgments of patients or doctors which had proved the undoing of its predecessors. (Kendell 1975a: 309)

As he reports, Scadding does not define 'biological disadvantage', but Kendell argues that it must involve increased mortality and reduced fertility, 'whether it should embrace other impairments as well is less obvious' (Kendell 1975a: 310). Thus, he uses this criterion to test the idea of mental illness:

> Do mental illnesses possess the essential attributes of illness or not? Do they, by reducing either fertility or life expectancy, produce a significant biological disadvantage? (Kendell 1975a: 311)

After some investigation—which turns on empirical facts about the effects of these putative illnesses—he is able to come to a modest, positive conclusion:

> Schizophrenia, manic depressive illness, and also some sexual disorders and some forms of drug dependence, carry with them an intrinsic biological disadvantage, and on these grounds are justifiably regarded as illness; but it is not clear whether the same is true of neurotic illness and the ill-defined territory of personality disorder. (Kendell 1975a: 315)

Three things are worth noting about Kendell's approach:

♦ He does not attempt to show that mental illnesses are illnesses because they are also, really, physical illnesses. He thus avoids one line of criticism expressed by Szasz. (Had he done so then Szasz would argue that he had merely shown the reality of some further physical illnesses.)

- His criterion of illness is general. It applies to physical and mental illness. Any condition is an illness if it leads to biological disadvantage of the right sort. If the definition of illness in general is correct, then the method promises to produce quite general and neutral answers without begging the question in favour of or against mental versus physical conditions. That said, it is originally derived from considerations of paradigmatic physical illnesses.

- The criterion is purely factual and value free. It is a matter simply of empirical fact whether a condition increases mortality and reduces fertility. If it does, then it is an illness. If not, then it is not. (Since the condition is a conjunction, strictly if merely one conjunct is satisfied that is not sufficient to count. Of course, it might plausibly be interpreted as a disjunction: increased mortality *or* reduced fertility.)

Kendell's approach faces a dilemma. On the one hand, he inherits from Scadding some ambiguity about what 'biological disadvantage' means; without some further explanation that will not shed light on the nature of mental illness. On the other hand, attempting to solve that problem by appeal to the idea of increased mortality and reduced fertility produces a substantial theory of illness or disease, but one that is vulnerable to the objection that it does not articulate what is essential to the idea of all illnesses. Roughly speaking, it seems plausible that one might be genuinely ill without this leading to increased mortality and reduced fertility. Whilst those measures might well address illnesses that, specifically, are life-threatening and undermine reproductive ability, neither risk seems to be an essential feature of everything that we might call 'illness' or 'disease'.

The US philosopher Christopher Boorse also attempts to articulate a value-free, purely descriptive account of disease but using a conceptually richer notion: that of biological function in general. He notes strategically that:

> Reluctance to require any analogy between mental and physical health tends to cripple clinical discussion, from high-level theory to the analysis of particular conditions like homosexuality. The reason is that mental-health theory and practice have not sprung up in a vacuum. On the contrary, they originally rose within physiological medicine, a mature and fairly well-articulated body of thought. From this established discipline they borrowed both the root notion of health and the many unspoken assumptions around it: that health is worth promoting, for example, and that well-informed observers ought in principle to agree on the norms of the healthy personality. (Boorse 1998: 108)

From this, Boorse argues that our understanding of mental health should be informed by root notions of health in general, drawn from physical medicine. This, in turn, leads him to frame a definition of health and illness, or rather disease in general in what he hopes will be value free terms (I will return to his distinction between illness and disease shortly).

An organism is healthy at any moment in proportion as it is not diseased; and a disease is a type of internal state of the organism which:

1) interferes with the performance of some natural function—i.e. some species-typical contribution to survival and reproduction—characteristic of the organism's age;

2) is not simply in the nature of the species, i.e. is either atypical of the species or, if typical, mainly due to environmental causes. (Boorse 1998: 108)

This analysis introduces a key extra concept compared with Kendell's broadly statistical model. Natural functions are *normative*. One can talk about the dispositions of an organism being in accord with them or not and, if not, one can talk of 'failures of function'. At the same time, descriptivist supporters of the use of natural functions claim that they are, nevertheless, purely descriptive and scientific terms. This will become increasingly important.

I hinted that Boorse, unlike Kendell, distinguishes between the concepts of disease and illness. Disease is supposed to be the more fundamental notion and value free. Illness is a disease that is 'serious enough to be incapacitating' and 'undesirable for its bearer' (Boorse 1975: 61).

Like any substantial philosophical definition, Boorse's account faces criticism. One key question concerns whether functions really can both capture the richer notion of normativity whilst also being rooted in purely descriptive science, to which I will return. But even on the assumption that functions can play that role, the kind of further difficulty the definition faces is summarised by the philosopher of psychiatry Rachel Cooper in a critical overview paper on recent definitions called 'Disease' (Cooper 2002). She points out the relevance of four different options in explaining:

For the function of X to be Z any of the following might be considered necessary:
1. X was originally selected because it does Z.
2. In the recent past selection has been responsible for maintaining X because it does Z.
3. Currently selection is responsible for maintaining X because it does Z.
4. At all times X has been selected because it does Z.
It is difficult to choose between these options as each is associated with potential problems. (Cooper 2002: 268)

One of the problems that Cooper highlights is that if one opts for the original selective advantages of some trait that, as a matter of fact, now also *prima facie* serves another function then failure of that current *prima facie* function will not count as disease. If, instead, recent history is taken to be key, then, because human societies and technologies now affect actual reproduction, traits that might seem *prima facie* to be dysfunctional, but are compensated for through human intervention, cannot count as diseases.

I will return to reassess the idea of failure of biological function when discussing Jerome Wakefield's model below, but before that it will be useful to put the debate between Szasz, on the one hand, and Kendell and Boorse, on the other, into a broader context. This is provided in an overview developed by Bill (KWM) Fulford.

## 2. **Putting the debate into context**

### Fulford's overview of the role of values in psychiatry

How can the disagreement between Szasz' values-based critique of psychiatry, and Kendell and Boorse's values-excluding defence be assessed? A useful perspective is provided by the psychiatrist and philosopher Bill Fulford. His analysis is a form of philosophical diagnosis. The significant feature of the debate, he argues, is not so much about what they *explicitly* disagree on, but on what they *implicitly* agree and disagree. Once this is highlighted, a different conclusion can be drawn. Taking Szasz and Kendell to represent the poles of the debate, Fulford argues that:

> Both authors assume that mental illness is the target problem: Szasz wants to 'raise the question, is there such a thing as mental illness'? Kendell, similarly, seeks to 'decide whether mental illnesses are legitimately so-called'. Both then turn to the concept of physical illness, acknowledging certain difficulties of definition, but suggesting criteria which they take to be self-evidently essential to its meaning: Szasz' criterion is 'deviation from the clearly defined norms of the structural and functional integrity of the body'. Kendell's is 'biological disadvantage, which must embrace both increased mortality and reduced fertility'. Finally, both return to mental illness. Szasz points out that for mental illness, the relevant norms of bodily structure and functioning are not available: on the contrary, he argues, the norms of mental illness are 'ethical, legal and social'. Kendell, on the other hand, draws on epidemiological and statistical data to show that many mental illnesses are biologically disadvantageous in his sense, being associated with reduced life and/or reproductive expectations. Hence by Szasz' criteria of physical illness, mental illness is a myth, whereas by Kendell's it is not. (Fulford 1999a: 169)

Both agree that mental illness is conceptually problematic. Both agree that physical illness is conceptually simple and also value free. They disagree on the details of the criteria they draw from physical illness, but their broader disagreement is then on how mental illness meets the criteria abstracted. Szasz argues that putative mental illnesses answer to evaluative norms and thus fail to meet the criteria for illness. Kendell argues that they fit his preferred criteria of increased mortality and decreased fertility.

With the lie of the land set out in this way, Fulford goes on to argue that Szasz, like his fellow anti-psychiatrists, is right to claim that mental illness is value-laden (see below for his reason). He is wrong, Fulford argues, to contrast mental illness, conceptually, with physical illness. Mental illness and physical illness are both value terms. This is not always noticed because mental illness appears to be more overtly value-laden than physical illness, but this appearance is a reflection of a property that the generic term illness, as a value term, shares with all other value terms (see below).

As I have summarised above, biologically-minded psychiatrists, such as Kendell and Boorse, argue, in supposed defence of psychiatry, that mental illness is, perhaps contrary to appearances, value-free and thus broadly comparable to physical illness. Fulford responds that, whilst they are right to compare mental and physical illness in this respect, they are wrong to assume that the scientific foundations of medicine (including psychiatry) depend on eliminating the evaluative elements. To the contrary, once their equal status as value terms is recognised, the scientific parts of medicine (to the extent that science itself is value free) can be demarcated.

So, what are Fulford's arguments? Fulford draws here particularly on the work of philosophers, such as R. M. Hare (1919–2002) and J. L. Austin (1911–1960), writing particularly in the middle decades of the 20th century in the Oxford 'school' of linguistic analytic philosophy. His method, in the opening chapter of his book, is somewhat like the therapeutic method of the philosopher Ludwig Wittgenstein (1889–1951). By providing a philosophical diagnosis of the source of the difficulty—assumptions made about the role of values in psychiatry and the comparison and contrast with physical illness—the temptation to misguided philosophical theorising falls away. As Wittgenstein puts it:

> The real discovery is the one which enables me to stop doing philosophy when I want to. The one that gives philosophy peace, so that it is no longer tormented by questions which bring *itself* into question. (Wittgenstein 1953: §133)

The key assumption that mistakenly drives both anti-psychiatry and biological defences of psychiatry is that physical illness is conceptually simple and value-free. This motivates the anti-psychiatrists to compare mental illness unfavourably with physical illness and it motivates defenders of psychiatry to attempt to argue that mental illness is, like physical illness, value-free. Without the assumption, however, neither mistaken argumentative move is necessary nor justified.

Having set the scene in this way, Fulford develops a substantial philosophical analysis of the full range of pathological concepts, both physical and mental. In the first third of his book, he examines what illnesses have in common and it is from this that he advances the claim that both mental illness and physical illness are value terms. In this, he draws particularly on Hare's early work, especially his *Language of Morals,* on the logical properties of value terms (Hare 1952).

Hare pointed out that the value *judgments* expressed by (or implicit in) value *terms* are made on the basis of criteria that, in themselves, are *descriptive* (or factual) in nature. The value judgment expressed by 'this is a good strawberry', in one of Hare's examples, is made on the basis that the strawberry in question is, as a matter of fact, 'sweet, grub-free'. Hare then points out that where the descriptive criteria for a given value judgment are widely agreed or settled upon, it is these *descriptive* criteria that may come to dominate the use of the value term in question. This is a simple consequence of repeated association. In the case of strawberries, most people in most contexts value (prefer, like, enjoy) strawberries that are sweet and grub-free. Hence, the use of 'good strawberry' comes to be associated with descriptions such as 'sweet, grub-free, etc.' to the extent that it is this *descriptive* meaning that becomes dominant in the use of the term. This contrasts with, say, pictures where there are no settled descriptive criteria for a good picture because there is no general agreement about pictorial aesthetics. Hare's general conclusion, therefore, is this: value terms by which *shared* values are expressed may come, by a process of simple association, to look like *descriptive* (or factual) terms, whereas value terms expressing values over which there is disagreement, remain overtly value-laden in use.

This general claim applies equally to medical language. If illness (generically) is a value term and if mental illness is more overtly value-laden than physical illness, this is neither because (as Szasz argued) mental illness is a moral, rather than a scientific concept, nor (as Kendell and Boorse argued) because psychiatric science is less advanced than the sciences in areas of physical medicine such as cardiology. Rather, Fulford argues, it is because psychiatry is concerned with areas of human experience and behaviour, such as emotion, desire, volition and belief, where people's values are particularly highly diverse. Following the Oxford philosopher J. L. Austin, Fulford distinguishes between problems of definition and problems of use to suggest that, whilst at heart mental and physical illness are both equally definitionally complex, mental illness is more problematic in use because it reflects more problematic areas of human experience and behaviour, namely areas such as emotion, desire, volition and belief, in which people's values tend to be highly diverse.

Although explicitly responding to Szasz' *Myth of Mental Illness,* Fulford does not himself present his work as a defence of the reality of mental illness so much as an exercise in what another Oxford philosopher, Gilbert Ryle, called 'logical geography'. He sets out to give an account of the logical geography of medicine, of the given features of the uses of the medical concepts. If medical terms are value terms, in Hare's sense, then many of the features of their use, including a detailed analysis of the many different kinds of disease concept, follow from the general logical properties they share with all value terms, combined, of course, with contingent features of human values (in particular the diversity of values in psychiatry).

Powerful as these (as Fulford puts it) 'off the shelf' arguments may be from philosophical value theory, there is clearly more to the meaning of the medical concepts than simply a (negative) value judgment, overt or implicit. In the latter two-thirds of *Moral Theory and Medical Practice*, Fulford, thus, moves from the general to the particular, seeking to develop an account of the particular kind of negative value by which, on this view, the medical concepts are characterised. Here, his general claim, advanced with some caution and the suggestion that there may be merely a family resemblance between different instances of illness (mental and physical), is that an explanation of the full range of uses of the medical concepts requires, in addition to the more familiar function-based accounts of disease, an agency-based account of patients' experiences of illness. The line of argument in this part of Fulford's book is to work, as it were, backwards from the phenomenological features of different kinds of illness experience to the hypothesis that the primary experience of illness is a particular kind of 'failure of ordinary doing' (Fulford 1989: 120).

Fulford draws here on Austin's account of agency and his characterisation of ordinary doing as the kind of action that one 'gets on and does' without having to try, without having intentions explicitly in mind (Austin 1957). A failure to be able to do this kind of thing, in the absence of external constraint, captures, Fulford argues, the somewhat paradoxical character of experiences of illness. As a hypothesis, moreover, it helps to explain a number of the key features of the logical geography of medicine. In particular, the idea that illness comprises an internally generated failure of ordinary doing explains its value-ladenness because the ineliminable concept of *failure* (of ordinary doing) itself suggests an ineliminable (negative) value judgement. This is true of physical illness, as well as of mental illness, but when it comes to mental illness, an agency-based account allows, as Fulford argues in detail, a more complete account than any function-based account, of the wide variety of different kinds of psychopathology as different kinds of failure in what Fulford, again explicitly adopting Austin's terminology, calls the 'machinery in action'.

Of course, an agency-based account of illness deserves to be questioned. Perhaps the most obvious criticism concerns the status of pain. Fulford points out that not all pain is constitutive of illness, only negatively evaluated pains, but this does not address the key question of how negatively evaluated pains are constitutive of illness on an action failure model. Here, Fulford's suggestion, drawing on his general approach of there being different parts of the overall machinery of action, is that 'pain is unlike movement in being something one does something *about*' (Fulford 1989: 137). Thus, a pain that one cannot 'do something about', specifically a pain from which one cannot withdraw in the absence of perceived preventing causes, is experienced as (a symptom of) illness. This move, it may be thought, does not place the suffering of pain sufficiently central in the analysis of illness. Indeed, Fulford argues, contrary to many others, that pain is *not* central to the *meaning* of illness. It is rather a contingent matter that pain has this particular role (of withdrawal from noxious stimuli) in the machinery of action.

There is a further aspect of Fulford's model worth mentioning. If illness, in general, can be unified through the idea of action failure, why is there a perceived difference in practice between mental and physical illness? Why, for example, is there an anti-psychiatry movement, but no anti-cardiology movement?

Part of Fulford's answer to this flows from the feature of the logic of values outlined above. There is general agreement about the values concerned in physical illness, but wide disagreement over those concerned in mental illness (again, broadly speaking).

In Chapter 2, I will describe how much of the directly practical impact of Fulford's work (in values-based practice) comes from his characterisation of psychiatry and mental health more widely, as being, in this sense, evaluatively complex, rather than, as many of psychiatry's supporters, as well as its critics have argued, scientifically deficient. However, a second part of Fulford's answer to the more problematic nature of psychiatry and mental health, is implicit in the latter part of *Moral Theory and Medical Practice*, in his shift from function-based analyses of disease to agency-based analyses of illness. Fulford's point is that while the two kinds of account, function-based and agency-based, are equivalent in explanatory power across many areas of pathology, only an agency-based account can explain the full range of uses of the concept at the very heart of *psycho*pathology, the clinical concept of delusion, and such an account brings with it essentially normative (and, hence, contestable) judgements of rationality.

## The status of the likeness argument

Whilst Fulford's analysis helps place the debate about mental illness in a new light—setting out the surface disagreement against an underlying background of shared assumptions—his own approach has itself, recently, been criticised. In his book *The Metaphor of Mental Illness* (Pickering 2006), the philosopher Neil Pickering attempts to diagnose why there is continuing disagreement about the status of mental illness despite careful analysis. He argues that this is, in part, because of shared dependence on what he calls the 'likeness argument' that, he argues, is fundamentally flawed.

According to Pickering, the likeness argument is supposed to resolve the status of mental illness by showing that putative mental illness is, indeed, sufficiently like illness. It does this in one of two ways. Either, it takes a paradigmatic form of illness, a specific case like hypertension or physical illness more generally, and shows that mental illness is sufficiently like it because it shares sufficient of its features, or it abstracts a generic concept of illness (again, typically from physical illness) and shows that mental illness fits sufficient features of that general concept to count as illness.

Pickering argues that Fulford's analysis shows a partial insight into this, but fails to appreciate that the lessons apply to his own account:

> Though Szasz and Kendell both recruit a paradigm likeness argument, Fulford notices that each calls upon different features of his chosen paradigm (physical illness) in order to prove his case. This explains, as Fulford neatly points out, why despite the fact that both use the likeness argument, they manage to reach opposite conclusions. As a result, neither can necessarily hope to convince the other, or any one else for that matter, and the radical question goes unresolved. This clearly presents a problem in using the paradigm version of the likeness argument, which is one of Fulford's principal points. However, it turns out that Fulford is not objecting to the likeness argument as such, for he too uses it … abstracting … a generic concept of illness (action failure) from paradigmatic physical examples of illness, and employing that to try and resolve the question of whether mental illness exists, by showing that action failure defines illness, and is a principal feature of conditions such as schizophrenia and alcoholism. (Pickering 2006: 16)

Why, then, does the likeness argument fail to settle the matter? Pickering argues that it depends on two assumptions both of which can be questioned. He says:

> If the likeness argument is to resolve this dispute, then two things must, I think, be taken to be the case:
> ♦ that there are features of human conditions such as schizophrenia, which decide what category, or kind, these conditions are a member of;
> ♦ that, with respect to the presence or absence of these features, a condition such as schizophrenia is describable independent of the category it is assigned to. (Pickering 2006: 17)

The first is a general condition derived from a view of how concepts apply to things. The suggestion is that concepts apply in virtue of conditions having objective features. This stands in contrast, for example, to a view where all such concept application depends on an imaginative human judgement. The second is a more specific assumption relevant to the debate about mental illness. It is that the ascription of features to conditions—putative illnesses—can be made independently of a top-down decision as to the illness-status of those conditions.

Pickering suggests that both assumptions can be questioned. Criticism of the first—which he calls the 'weak objection' to the likeness argument—typically depends on pressing the role of human interests and values in the formation of human concepts. Nevertheless, as he goes on to concede, for the moment at least, there need be no incompatibility between acknowledging a role for interests and values in setting up a scheme of concepts and its autonomous application. (One direct way to get an objection off the ground would be to subscribe to a form of constructionism about concepts criticised in Chapter 4 of this book.)

The 'strong objection' turns on questioning the second assumption. Pickering argues that the ascription of features to conditions—putative illnesses—depends on the overall category—illness or not—into which they are placed. The argument for this is piecemeal. In each of three cases— alcoholism, attention deficit hyperactivity disorder (ADHD), schizophrenia— he offers competing descriptions of their basic features manifesting first an assumption that they are illnesses and second that they are not. The behavioural features of alcoholism, for example, can equally be described in terms of moral weakness or of causally determined pathological behaviour. The same data can be equally well interpreted in the light of opposing top-down theories. Arguing that this is a general feature of such contested cases, Pickering concludes that the features themselves cannot be used to determine to which overall category the condition belongs. (He goes on to note that this claim also undermines the first assumption and thus his earlier concession was temporary.)

This criticism is, however, not as successful as Pickering suggests. His central claim is that detectable and observable features of a condition, a putative illness, cannot be described without begging the question of the pathological status of that condition. This is not, however, a surprising claim. If the correct description of the features is taken to imply a pathological status then, trivially, it cannot be independent of the overall status. Even if it merely provides evidential support, Pickering has really only undermined a foundationalist version of the likeness argument, one in which observational data can be established independently of any broader theoretical perspectives. But most accounts of scientific theories now accept the theory dependence of data and an essential holism in theory testing. Most would reject a foundational approach to data, as Pickering himself later reports (Pickering 2006: 167).

Rejecting foundationalism in favour of scientific holism does not show that the likeness argument (or some version of the likeness argument) cannot work as part of a broader investigation of illness, which is the way, for example, Fulford suggests his own investigation is intended: as an investigation of the 'logical geography' of the medical concepts rather than a metaphysical defence of mental illness (see above and also Chapter 5 for discussion of such a defence). Indeed, it is hard to see what could be wrong with the likeness argument itself, given its triviality. (If the possession of a particular kind of characteristic implies illness status and if a condition has a characteristic of that kind, then it is an illness.) It is surely only when it is combined with foundationalist assumptions that the broader argument is substantial, though flawed. (The substance involved in using a likeness argument as a piece of holism is provided not by the argument's logical form, but by the choice that is made as to the features that justify the application of the term 'illness'.)

Nor does rejecting foundationalism amount to the stronger claim Pickering sometimes makes expressed in passages such as:

> The causal and dysfunctional features of schizophrenia and alcoholism are *created* in the light of the kind of thing they are thought to be (Pickering 2006: 7, italics added)

> The relevant features of alcoholism *do not*, contrary to what it demands, *exist* independently of the category into which alcoholism is placed. (Pickering 2006: 27, italics added)

These are radical constitutive claims that amount to a form of idealism about mental and behavioural features. The holism that Pickering highlights only establishes an epistemological point: that we cannot *establish* or *know* the nature of the features of a condition independently of establishing or knowing an overall classification. This is not the same as saying that the features are *constituted* as the features they are through human judgement.

So something akin to the likeness argument that Pickering protests against is still possible with the proviso that it is not thought of as a kind of foundational project. Judgements about mental and behavioural features, and overall judgements about conditions, form part of a larger package of ideas which have to be judged as a whole.

## 3. A biological teleological model of mental illness

With Fulford's and Pickering's diagnostic accounts in place, I will now turn to a final substantive analysis of mental illness. The US philosopher Jerome Wakefield has outlined an alternative to the analysis of Fulford, which shares Fulford's aim to reconcile a role for both values and facts.

Unlike Boorse and Kendell, Wakefield does not attempt to provide a value-free analysis of disease, but he suggests, as others have argued before him, that the medical concepts can be analysed into a value element combined with a value-free medical science core, itself 'anchored in evolutionary theory' (Wakefield 1999: 465). He calls this a 'harmful dysfunction analysis'. It contrasts with Fulford's analysis in that, in the latter, facts and values mingle 'all the way down'. (Note that, although, perhaps influenced by Boorse, Wakefield talks of 'disorder', rather than 'illness' or 'disease'—he avoids the challenge of distinguishing between them. Indeed, he comments: 'some writers draw distinctions among *disorder, disease,* and *illness. Disorder* is perhaps the broader term because it covers traumatic injuries as well as disease/illness. I ignore these differences' (Wakefield 1992: 374).)

At the heart of the value-free core is the notion of a failure of biological function (of which more below), but Wakefield does not attempt a completely 'values out' analysis. Illnesses, or as he calls them disorders, are *harmful* failures of function. This helps encode the practical aims of medicine to intervene in particular cases. Nevertheless, Wakefield's central aim is to characterise a purely descriptive *core* for medical science using the idea of biological functions.

The challenge of giving a descriptive, non-evaluative account of function to explain illness is to give an account of *failure* of function. Only if an account can be given of what a *divergence* of the behaviour of a system from its function comprises has the notion of a function which could be successfully *or* unsuccessfully executed been substantiated. If such an account of function could be given in value-free, descriptive terms, then it would *ipso facto* successfully account for failure of function. Thus, it would be a mistake to assume that in characterising disorder partly as a *failure* of function, Wakefield has already conceded the game to value theorists because 'failure' is an evaluative concept. If function could be analysed in descriptive terms then so could failure of function. An evaluative concept would be reduced to a value-free descriptive analysis.

It may still seem that, in the case of function, a descriptive account is a hopeless non-starter precisely because the distinction between success and failure surely cannot be reduced to a purely factual or descriptive vocabulary. Just such a descriptivist account of natural function has, however, been proposed in the philosophy of language and thought. Ruth Millikan proposes that the intentionality or 'aboutness' of thoughts and beliefs can be naturalised using the notion of biological functions (see especially Millikan 1984). She argues that even conscious human purposes are susceptible to this form of reductionist naturalism (Millikan 1998: 309).

Much has been written (by Millikan and others) on the definition of biological function. Roughly speaking, however, it is that function that a particular trait of an organism exemplifies, and explains the evolutionary success and survival value of that trait. Crucially, biological functions are distinct from dispositions.

The biological function of a trait and its dispositions can diverge. Engineering limitations might cause the actual behavioural dispositions of a trait to diverge from the biological function it thus only partially exemplifies. The divergences might themselves be life-threatening and play no positive part in explaining the value of the trait. The best explanation of the survival of that organism and those like it cites the *function* that helped propagation or predator evasion, for example, and not those aspects of its behavioural dispositions that diverged unhelpfully from it.

This point is sometimes put by saying that what matters is not which traits or dispositions are selected, but what *function* they are selected *for*. The distinction between 'selection of' and 'selection for' can be illustrated by the example of a child's toy (Sober 1984). A box allows objects of different shapes to be posted into it through differently shaped slots in the lid. The round slot thus allows the insertion of balls, for example. It may be that the actual balls allowed through or 'selected' in one case are all green, but they are selected *for* their round cross-section, not their green colour. Millikan stresses the fact that the biological function of a trait may be displayed in only a minority of actual cases. It is the function of sperm to fertilise an egg, but the great majority of sperm fails in this regard (Millikan 1984: 34).

Since biological functions can diverge from mere dispositions, they have extra resources necessary for accounting for *failure* of function. The distinction between success and failure of a system, organism or organ can be defined by reference to its functioning in accord with its biological function.

Wakefield's work on mental illness is in the same tradition: providing a reductionist account of a problematic concept by appeal to evolutionary theory. He offers an initially distinct, but eventually similar, account of natural functions. Drawing on essentialist accounts of natural kinds, such as water or gold, he suggests that natural functions likewise have an underlying essence. Thus, natural functions are defined as sharing whatever the initially unknown essential process is, which explains prototypical non-accidental beneficial effects such as eyes seeing. This is a surprising claim given that what unites natural kinds such as gold or water are first order physical properties. No first order physical properties unite natural functions, but Wakefield goes on to invoke explanation and natural selection in a much more standard way:

> A natural function of a biological mechanism is an effect of the mechanism that explains the existence, maintenance or nature of the mechanism via the same essential process (whatever it is) by which prototypical non-accidental beneficial effects ... explain the mechanism which cause them ... It turns out that the process that explains the prototypical non-accidental benefits is natural selection acting to increase inclusive fitness of the organism. (Wakefield 1999: 471–2)

Thus, like Millikan, Wakefield relies on an account of natural function drawn from explanation within evolutionary theory to distinguish those dispositions that accord with a system's naturally selected function from those which do not.

Having briefly sketched the typical form of a descriptivist account of natural function, I will now turn to recent criticism of it by both Bill Fulford and the Aristotelian philosopher Christopher Megone. Both critics share the view that Wakefield's account of function cannot escape an evaluative element that resists reduction to descriptive terms. Whilst I agree with the thrust of their attack, I will argue that further work would have to be done to show that it is *values* that cause this problem.

In a lengthy commentary on Wakefield's work, Bill Fulford attempts to eliminate all terms that are either apparently value-based or 'genuinely' teleological from Wakefield's definition of failure of function. His aim is to show that this task fails and, thus, that Wakefield fails to reduce the concept of function to austere descriptive terms. Thus, the main weight of Fulford's argument occurs as he discusses the final variation. Here, he makes two suggestions. One is that:

> [I]f organisms, as distinct from rocks and winds, have purposes, then, in addition to the causal language of evolution, we can (non-metaphorically) speak of them teleologically ... The nonmetaphorical use of teleological as well as causal language of organisms is not as such anti-scientific... All the same the necessity for teleological... language in this context directly conflicts with Wakefield's express aim of establishing a purely causal theory. And this aim ... in turn reflects the fact that teleological language—purposes, intentions, motives, means and ends—is, from the point of view of a conventional picture of science, uncomfortably close to values. (Fulford 1999b: 416)

Without some further argument, however, this point is not decisive. Wakefield is following the tradition of attempting to 'naturalise' purposive talk by showing how it is really disguised purely causal talk. He does this through the idea that natural selection can underpin a definition of function which is not evaluative. If this were successful it would enable him to talk of biological functions or purposes and thus failures of function, secure in the knowledge that this were merely a shorthand for an austere description of underlying causal processes. (Millikan wishes to use just such an account to reduce conscious human purposes and intentions.) This is not to say that Wakefield (or Millikan) is *successful* in this reduction, but something more is needed to indicate that this appeal to natural selection fails.

Fulford also suggests (admittedly expressed as a conditional 'if ...') that 'purpose implies a positive value judgement' (Fulford 1999b: 417). If this were the case then reductionism to purely descriptive causal language would fail, but it is far from clear that the concept of natural or biological function implies a positive value judgement. To investigate this point further I will turn to Megone's criticism.

Megone provides a distinct argument against Wakefield's descriptive account of function as follows:

> According to Wakefield, on this model, 'the heart exists for the purpose of pumping the blood in the sense that past hearts having this effect causally explains how hearts came to exist and be maintained in the species and the genesis of the heart's detailed structure' (Wakefield 2000: 31). The most basic difficulty here is that past hearts' pumping the blood figure in all sorts of causal stories, stories in which agents die young, or agents do not reproduce, or agents reproduce but defectively, and so on. It is not the case that hearts pumping the blood have simply caused hearts to exist. So hearts pumping the blood does not causally explain how hearts came to exist. This cannot therefore be the sense in which the pumping of the blood is a functionally explicable activity of the heart. (Megone 2000: 60–1)

Whilst there is something right about this objection, it is noticeable that Megone runs together causal *explanation* and mere causal *relations*. By contrast, Wakefield, like Millikan, relies on specifying the function of systems through what best explains their continued existence. Thus, he can reply that the divergent causal *relations* do not *explain* the heart's existence. Recall again the distinction between the dispositions of a system and its natural function. Its dispositions are genuine causal consequences of the system's nature, but do not explain its existence. Before returning briefly to assess the prospects for this naturalistic reduction of function, I will turn first to an explicitly value based account. Must function presuppose value?

## A teleological account of function?

Megone goes on to propose an alternative, irreducibly teleological, account of function, which shares Fulford's emphasis on positive evaluation of goals:

> The fundamental idea is that the heart's function must be a goal, good from some perspective, and pumping the blood can be seen as achieving a goal if that activity contributes to the persistence of the species, and that in turn is, from some perspective, good ... The evaluative account of 'function' only holds that if the activity of a member of a natural kind, or of its part, is to be open to functional explanation there must be *some perspective* from which that activity is seen as good. Only from that perspective is the behaviour functionally explicable. (Megone 2000: 57)

This open-ended talk of there being 'some perspective' is meant to respond to cases (mentioned by Wakefield) where functional explanations are offered by theorists who do not *themselves* positively value the outcome they invoke, such as the idea that social welfare policy has the function of controlling, rather than helping, the poor or that parts of harmful viruses can be function-ally explained. Hence, Megone goes on '(o)f course functional explanation of the behaviour of parts will be possible in the cases above if it is said, for example, that the survival of the virus ... is good in the sense that it is good ... for that kind itself' (Megone 2000: 57–8).

So although Megone argues that systems can only be given functional explanation if there exists merely *some perspective* from which that activity is *seen as good*, he goes on to argue that that perspective is an essential part of the explanation. It is not arbitrary *who* it is that positively values the outcome.

In fact, more needs to be said than this about the connection between positive value and such a model of an irreducible teleological explanation. To explore this further I will briefly summarise an account of teleology developed elsewhere by another value theorist: the philosopher Mark Bedau (Bedau 1998). My purpose in describing his account is first to try to make more explicit the role that values might play in a genuinely teleological account of function and then to assess the consequences that this has for reductionist, descriptivist accounts of biological function like Wakefield's and Millikan's.

Like Fulford and Megone, Bedau rejects attempts to sanitise teleology through an austere descriptive account, dismissing, for example, Boorse (Bedau 1998: 261), and develops, instead, an explicitly value-based account. He does this by describing a three-fold hierarchy of 'telic' structures (grades G1, G2, G3), arguing that only one of them (G3) is genuinely teleological. Bedau defines the first grade of telic structure thus:

> Where A is an agent who does something or has some property, B, in order to bring about some end C:
> (G1) A B's in order to C *iff* A B's and A's Bing contributes to Cing and Cing is good for A. (Bedau 1998: 267)

This does *not* give the form of teleological explanation. As Bedau points out, one may, for example, swim and one's swimming may contribute to one's fitness, but this may *not* be *why* one swims. It may not *explain* it. Similarly, it is a good thing for medical science that the beating of the heart makes a noise, but that is not *why* it beats. It does not explain its beating. What needs to be added to G1 is an explanatory connection ('because') between Bing and Cing, but there are two choices for the scope of that connection. Hence, there are two further telic grades:

> (G2) A B's in order to C *iff* (A B's *because* A's Bing contributes to Cing) and Cing is good for A ...
> (G3) A B's in order to C *iff* A B's *because* (A's Bing contributes to Cing and Cing is good for A) (Bedau 1998: 269)

To see why structure G2 is insufficient for genuine teleological explanation, consider three further examples which Bedau gives:

◆ Imagine a stick caught, initially by chance, against a rock in a flowing river, which creates a backwash that keeps the stick caught against the rock, creating the backwash. Although this case involves an effect of the system that explains the maintenance of the system (compare with the first part of Wakefield's definition quoted above), it is not an instance of teleology and fits none of G1–3. The stick does not create the backwash *in order* to stay against the rock.

- Now, imagine the stick replaced by an unconscious man caught against a rock, upstream from perilous falls. This example fits G2 because there is an explanatory relation between being stuck on the rock and creating a backwash, and it is also the case that being stuck on the rocks is good for the person concerned, but in fact the unconscious man does not create the backwash *in order* to remain stuck on the rocks. Thus, this is still not a case for teleological explanation.

- Finally, imagine a case where a conscious man deliberately moves himself into the same position, creating a backwash, because he positively values being stuck on the rock (so as not to go over the falls). This is a case of genuine goal-directed teleological explanation. It fits G3.

Bedau concludes that only the wide scope of G3 gives the logical form of genuine teleological explanation.

## So can biological function be reduced?

Does explanation by natural selection fit this form? Bedau argues not for the following reason:

> [I]n biological systems natural selection produces survival-promoting selection processes that explain why creatures have survival-promoting features. And survival is surely a good for living creatures, indeed, a paramount good. But natural selection also operates in certain populations of non-living entities and explains certain of their features ... Now, in contrast with forms of life, survival is neither good nor bad for non-living things ... So, natural selection over non-living populations is not a good-producing but merely a survival-producing process, and such a situation would exhibit *no* grades of teleology. (Bedau 1998: 281–2)

What are the consequences of Bedau's analysis of teleology for the debate about mental illness? First, it suggests that more has to be added to Megone's invocation of value in teleological explanation to rule out cases in which a valued end is present, but where teleological explanation is inappropriate. Secondly, it suggests one way in which there could be something right about Fulford's brief comment that genuine teleology is uncomfortably close to values. One might simply adopt something like Bedau's account as a stipulative definition of genuinely teleological explanation, thus ensuring the presence of a positively evaluated goal. Thirdly, it suggests that values are *not* in fact the key objection for reducing talk of functions to descriptions.

The reason for this last claim is that it is open to descriptivists just as much as to their opponents to accept the stipulation suggested in the second point above. If so, then they will have to concede that biological explanation is not 'genuinely teleological', since it does not involve covert appeal to values. However, they can argue that it was precisely one of the intellectual achievements of Darwinism to show how it is that apparently genuine teleological features in nature are really the result of non-teleological causal processes. So the concession is merely terminological and does not undermine the project of giving a naturalistic analysis of biological function.

If this diagnosis of the nature of the debate is correct then the primary disagreement should not be whether the concept of function is evaluative, but the more general issue of whether it can be reduced to the austere descriptive terms of the realm of law, to repeat the phrase I introduced at the start of the chapter. To repeat, if it could be shown that values could not be eliminated from an account of natural function then that would imply the falsity of reductionist naturalism, but that is not necessary to undermine reductionism. Whilst genuine teleology might presuppose values, there seems no reason to believe that biological functions do. (Recall that the fact that in characterising the goal of such reductionist naturalism, talk of '*failures* of function' does not concede the game to value theorists. It simply shows the scale of the problem for reductionism.) Thus, in the specific case of function, the debate need not be construed as most fundamentally 'values in' versus 'values out', but rather reductionism versus anti-reductionism.

Seen in this light, I think that reductionist naturalism still fails, and thus the aim of a plainly factual or austere descriptive causal account of natural function cannot be met. To see why, think again about the distinction between the mere dispositions and natural functions. As Megone correctly points out, there are diverse causal consequences of biological systems corresponding to its dispositions under different circumstances. What singles out its proper function is what *best explains* the continued existence of the system. It is this that provides the determinacy that underpins the distinction between behaviour which accords with proper function and that which does not. But this notion of best explanation is not like explanation in the realm of law. It is not like explaining an event by subsuming it under a law of nature as the acceleration of an object due to gravity might be explained. Rather, it turns on seeing a particular kind of explanatory pattern in the myriad causal relations that goes beyond the resources of nomological explanation. The realm of law lacks the resources to select between different dispositions as being correct or incorrect.

This point can be emphasised by recalling the distinction between what is selected and what it is selected for. The biological function is identified only with the latter, but to identify that function requires an interpretation that goes beyond the data of evolutionary success. One might try to put this point by saying that whilst the function that the dispositions and behaviour of a biological system partially exemplifies has to be *consistent* with that behaviour, it is not *determined* by it. In fact, however, the function does not even have to be consistent with the behaviour, because the behaviour only *partially* exemplifies the function. There may be engineering limitations that prevent the system successfully tracking the function, but given that the causal transactions of evolutionary history provide some constraint on the ascription of function, there are still an infinite number of different functions that meet that constraint. Consider, for example, all the functions that only diverge at a still future date. Systems with those functions would have been just as successful in the past.

What rules out these divergent functions is the pattern of explanation that we find natural in the context of evolutionary theory, but that pattern, although characteristic of evolutionary biology, finds no echo in the patterns found in the more basic science of the realm of law. Thus, the hope of grounding the one form of explanation in the more austere vocabulary of the realm of law cannot be successful.

To say this is to agree with the *conclusion* of value theorists who argue that no austere descriptive or plainly factual account of function can be given because that concept has a feature missing from any proposed reducing account given in purely causal and descriptive terms. The function that best explains the existence or maintenance of a system or trait turns, in part, on our perceptions of naturalness and salience in this context which differs from the patterns of explanation in physical science. These underpin our account of biological function in the light of causal dispositions. In other words, they underpin the distinction between certain ways of going on as according with a function and others that are merely part of the causal order which do not accord with that function. However, without further argument, there is no need to assume that this perceived pattern need be based either on values or goods.

To say this is to suggest that value theorists are looking in the wrong place for the presence of implicit values. Whilst biological function does not reduce to the language of physics, and not because it is genuinely teleological, this is *not* to say that the concept of illness can be built up in the following way: first take a non-evaluative, albeit explanatorily rich, concept of function and then add a further value component, such as harm. One difficulty for that project, which should have become clearer in this brief account, is that failure of function on Millikan's account is widespread. Because biological function is not equated with behavioural dispositions (such as dispositions under normal or even ideal circumstances), the *actual* dispositions of systems could always differ from the function, which explains their continued existence. This makes the prospect of identifying illness even with only the harmful instances of failure of function, as Wakefield suggests, unpromising.

## 4. Mild cognitive impairment: a case study in philosophy of psychiatry

How does the analysis of mental illness in general impact on an understanding of particular mental illnesses. In the final section of this chapter I will consider, as a case study, mild cognitive impairment (MCI). The central issue that will be raised is the connection between the pathological status of a condition and what I will term the 'plain facts' about the frequency and nature of its symptoms. In the case of MCI, the philosophical discussion will reveal that there are difficult judgements underpinning the status of the condition. Even if one can select a favoured general model of mental illness, that is no guarantee that it will generate easy answers in all cases.

MCI raises a number of *ethical* questions that have been discussed recently. Central, perhaps, is the concern that a diagnosis carries negative repercussions that might outweigh the more narrowly medical advantages of an early diagnosis, but whilst that concern may be appropriate, such ethical complications are a danger of any psychiatric classification or diagnosis, even the most well grounded. Any psychiatric diagnosis can carry a danger of stigma, for example.

What seems to make such ethical concerns more serious in this case is the implicit further concern that MCI is not a real, objective or, to use a more medical term, valid category or classification. If it is not valid, then any negative connotations of the diagnosis will not be outweighed by medical technological achievements. In other words, the further ethical issues are given much greater weight if the question of validity is not satisfactorily resolved.

The question of the reality, objectivity or validity of MCI can be subdivided into two issues:

- Is MCI a real, objective or valid feature of psychological phenomenology?
- Is MCI a real, objective or valid psychological illness, disease or pathology?

A condition might be a real, objective or valid feature of psychological phenomenology without being a real illness. It might be some other aspect of human living. Szasz suggests that this is the case with mental illness as a whole. Less controversially, the unusual ability to calculate, mentally and in a flash, the date of future Easter Sundays is a genuine feature of human living—some people possess the ability even if most do not—without either it, or its lack, being an illness. Being real as an illness is a very specific kind of being.

It is this, I suggest, that raises difficulties in the case of MCI by contrast with the easier question of whether something is a genuine feature of human living in some other way.

In a clinically informed philosophical discussion of MCI Lynne Corner, a researcher into psychosocial and cultural aspects of ageing, and John Bond, professor of social gerontology, usefully suggest that the question of whether MCI is real is made more difficult by an ambiguity in the sense of the word 'normal'. They suggest that whilst 'physiological and cognitive decline is assumed to be a normal experience', this still leaves 'boundary problems' about 'distinguishing "normal ageing" from "disease"' (Corner and Bond 2006: 3–4). Thus, if the symptoms of MCI are continuous with the ordinary phenomena of physiological and cognitive decline then they might also be merely normal, but this does not settle the status of MCI because 'normal' can mean either: 'normative, i.e. usual, or it can mean non-pathological' (Corner and Bond 2006: 4).

On the assumption that MCI is at least continuous with phenomena that are 'normal' then its symptoms might be normal in the sense of usual but nevertheless pathological: an inevitable illness. Or they might be usual and non-pathological, merely a feature of ageing that, whilst regrettable, lacks the connotations of illness (for example, the appropriateness, if not the possibility, of treatment). (In principle on the assumption in play—that the symptoms of MCI are normal—they might be unusual but non-pathological akin, for example, to an improved ability to solve crosswords with age which might affect a small lucky proportion of the population. Perhaps such a crossword puzzler might be reassured by their doctor: 'Well that is very unusual but there is no need to worry: it is not a symptom of any illness. You are perfectly normal.')

Thus, the question: 'Is MCI a normal feature of ageing or not?' is, as Corner and Bond point out, ambiguous between these two interpretations of 'normal'. They themselves go on to characterise the first sense—the mere statistics, as it were—using the term 'normative' ('normative, i.e. usual') and this contrasts with the sense of non-pathological. Whilst that is a perfectly valid use of the term 'normative', I wish to stress a different sense of it that is distinct from the merely statistically usual. This is the sense of normative connected with a distinction between correctness and incorrectness. This second sense of 'normative' will help shed light on the second sense of 'normal' mentioned above, the sense of non-pathological. I hope to tie the distinction between pathological and non-pathological to the distinction between correctness and incorrectness. I hope that this will help illustrate the way in which MCI nicely exemplifies some of the issues about the objectivity of medical classification.

It is useful to consider two analogical cases: from philosophy of language and moral philosophy. In the philosophy of language, especially in work influenced by the later Wittgenstein, 'normative' is used to mark a *contrast* with the merely statistically usual. In that field, it is used to mark the contrast between how a word *should* be used, determined by its meaning, and how, as a matter of fact, it *is* used, including incorrectly, but the distinction then prompts a puzzle.

A description of actual usage looks like the only description of the plain facts of the matter available. A careful examination of the phenomena of linguistic usage made, for example, by visiting Martian anthropologists (or anyone else occupying a position of 'cosmic exile' in Quine's memorable phrase (Quine 1960: 275)) would surely restrict itself to an analysis of the frequency and so forth with which words are used. The facts about how a word *should* be used look to be mysterious—and unavailable to the Martians—by comparison. So what is the relation between the two? How can an account of how a word should be used be derived or extracted from plain facts available? How can the normative features of linguistic use be explained in terms of descriptions of actual use?

These questions mirror a challenge from another area of philosophy: moral philosophy or ethics. The parallel question in moral philosophy is: how can one derive a moral 'ought' from an 'is'? Given an account, for example, of human customs—which lie etymologically behind the word 'moral'—how can one extract not just an account of what *is* done, but a conception of what *should* be done? Martian anthropologists look to be similarly challenged on this front. There is a philosophical tradition going back to David Hume that takes for granted the impossibility of any such derivation or reduction.

Although influential, the broad distinction between normative and non-normative claims is not without critics. The US philosopher John Searle, for example, attempts to show that one can derive an 'ought' from an 'is', and thus undermine one expression of the distinction. He frames an argument to a claim about how someone ought to act, from a supposedly value-free description that someone has uttered some words, via the claim that they have thereby undertaken a promise (Searle 1967). Anticipating potential objections, Searle attempts to make explicit all the further necessary stages but tries to ensure that each is merely descriptive. However, as Hare argues in reply, the eventual argument still requires for its validity that one accepts a prescriptive principle that one ought to keep one's promises (Hare 1967). Hare effectively exposes an implicit prescriptive premise that is necessary for Searle's argument to work.

More recently, Hilary Putnam has criticised the 'dichotomy' of fact and value (Putnam 2002). His requirements for such a dichotomy are, however, substantial. He suggests that a dichotomy has to place all cases to be sorted on one side or the other, that philosophical problems are quickly solved once the dichotomy is applied, and that both sides form natural kinds, that is, they both involve an essential unifying property (Putnam 2002: 10).

Putnam goes on to illustrate these requirements using a metaphysical distinction found in Hume and his later positivist followers, between facts—which were claimed to be *picturable* in true thoughts and sentences—and values which were not. On this family of accounts, facts make up the fabric of the world, whilst values merely depend on a projection from human subjectivity. As Putnam plausibly highlights, however, there is good reason to deny both the underlying metaphysical picture and the dichotomy it motivates. One objection turns on the impossibility of factoring out the descriptive and factual from the prescriptive aspects of 'thick' moral concepts, such as 'crime' or 'cruel', as though their application in judgements depended on recognising only the descriptive aspects and then superimposing a further prescription. In this he draws on the work of McDowell (McDowell 1998b: 198–218). (It is worth noting the *ad hominum* point that, whilst McDowell criticises any such attempt to disentangle descriptive and prescriptive aspects of 'thick' value judgements, he does not deny an important distinction between what is normative and what is not.)

Putnam does, however, concede that there can be a distinction if not a dichotomy: 'there is a distinction to be drawn (one that is useful in some contexts) between ethical judgments and other sorts of judgements … *But nothing metaphysical follows from the existence of a fact value distinction in this modest sense*' (Putnam 2002: 19). This is enough of a distinction, however, for my purposes.

The case of Searle and Putnam suggests that it is important to distinguish a semantic claim—a claim about the meaning of fact and value terms—and a metaphysical claim about the reality of values.

- The semantic thesis is that normative claims cannot be analysed into non-normative claims.
- The metaphysical thesis is that only non-normative claims can characterise the fabric of the world, of outer reality.

I will assume, in what follows, that a proper response to Searle and Putnam is to maintain the former but reject the latter.

To return to MCI, if we take 'normal' to mean normative in the sense that is distinct from what is merely statistically usual, it suggests a different way of focusing on the question of whether MCI is a valid diagnostic category. Whatever the 'plain facts' of the phenomenology of human ageing, there is a further question as to whether MCI is pathological. The analogy with the philosophy of language and with ethics suggests that there is a significant gap between the plain facts associated with physiological and cognitive decline, and the normative status of MCI. In other words, just as there seems to be a gap between saying that something is the case and saying that something ought to be the case, which itself mirrors the gap between saying how words (as a matter of fact) are used and saying how they must (normatively) be used in order to accord with their meaning, so too there seems to be a gap between biological facts to do with ageing and normative concerns about MCI. These analogies, however, prompt two questions:

◆ What is it about pathology that connects with normativity in this sense? In other words, how does the analogy with the normative status of correct linguistic usage or a morally appropriate action actually work?

◆ If the analogy does hold, then how can we answer the question of whether MCI is pathological (rather than merely fairly unusual)?

As outlined so far in this chapter, there are a number of positive answers to the first question. All 'values in' positions in the debate about mental illness stress a normative aspect of mental illness that flows from the presence of values. In different ways this view is shared by, for example, Szasz, Fulford and Nordenfelt, although they draw different conclusions from it (Szasz 1968; Fulford 1989; Nordenfelt 1995). This approach, however, requires that a connection can be established between diagnosis and what is recognisably a value.

In some cases, there does seem to be a close connection between DSM categories and a morally evaluative term. (The DSM-IV diagnosis of antisocial personality disorder includes reference to 'conning others for personal profit or pleasure' where 'conning' is clearly a moral value-laden term.) In other cases the nature of the value is less clear cut. (The same DSM category includes 'failure to conform to social norms'. Whilst 'failure' may be a morally evaluative term in this case, it is less clearly so.)

In *Moral Theory and Medical Practice*, Bill Fulford talks of 'a particular kind of value, medical or pathological value as distinct from, e.g., moral and aesthetic' (Fulford 1989: 215). There is, however, a danger in distinguishing medical values too sharply from more familiar kinds. It threatens to weaken the key claim that medical diagnosis is evaluative. If medical values were utterly distinct from other kinds of values and were simply defined as what guide medical diagnosis then the claim that such diagnosis is evaluative would be tautological.

Fulford, however, traces the evaluative element in the meanings of the medical concept directly to the *failure* of ordinary doing from which his general agency-based account of the widely different kinds of illness (bodily as well as mental) is derived. This, in turn, allows him to provide detailed piecemeal accounts of the moral and other evaluative connotations of particular medical terms, which address this concern in particular cases.

However, as I have argued above, there is a subtly different reason for thinking that diagnosis might be normative without necessarily being based on values. This stems from a response to Wakefield's descriptive account of mental disorder based on the concept of biological function. The function need not be a *usual* aspect of the behaviour of a trait, but rather is what best explains the continuance of that trait. Nevertheless, such explanation turns precisely on a transition from 'plain facts' to the normative status of an explanation given in terms of function. What makes that transition possible is a grasp of what would be a good reason for the trait and that is a normative notion: an aspect of the space of reasons rather than the realm of law.

In other words, the kind of explanation deployed in post-Darwinian accounts of biological functions shares something with the explicitly teleological 'just so stories' that they are designed to supplant. They both rely on notions of what is a good explanation, a good reason for something, over and above what is statistically likely. The function of a biological trait may correspond to something that is, statistically, unusual, but nevertheless explanatorily very powerful. If so, explanation in terms of biological function presupposes aspects of the space of reasons, rather than explaining them, and thus presupposes, rather than explains, its normativity.

Whilst the debate about the normative nature of psychiatric diagnosis is still in a state of flux, there is at least reason to think that the inference from plain facts to normative pathological status is problematic. This leads to the second question. How can the difficult judgement about the putative pathological status of MCI be guided? Is MCI pathological?

It may seem, however, that there is a way of escaping this difficult judgement. One route concerns whether MCI is a predictor 'that an individual will subsequently develop Alzheimer's Disease or dementia' (ibid: 4). Is it 'a transitional state between the cognition of normal ageing and mild dementia' (ibid: 4)? Assume, for a moment, that it transpires that there is such a connection and, thus, that MCI can be used to predict Alzheimer's Disease. We now also know that Alzheimer's is associated with the formation of amyloid plaques and neurofibrillary tangles in the brain. And thus it might seem that these connections are sufficient to escape the need for the difficult judgement. The objectivity of MCI is underpinned by its predictive validity: the connection to Alzheimer's and that, in turn, is underpinned by a developing patho-physiological account of brain changes that explain the associated mental symptoms. Those changes seem to be a plainly factual. Given the connections then the pathological status of MCI is justified.

Whilst the account of Alzheimer's does not suggest the practical difficulties of MCI—Alzheimer's is not often cited for critical attack by the anti-psychiatry movement—it does, nevertheless, depend on a difficult judgement of its own. The descriptions of amyloid plaques and neurofibrillary tangles do not wear their pathological statuses on their sleeves, any more than any merely unusual feature would. Rather, it is because of the putative explanatory connection between them and something that is independently identified as pathological that such physiological factors can seem to be a short cut to a difficult judgement. (This is an instance of the main problem for the likeness argument that Pickering highlights (see above).) Given that that normative judgement has already been made in some cases, then it is possible in other cases to side step explicitly normative judgements in favour of mere descriptions of the plain facts of brain structure. What makes these relevant, however, is the connection already established between them and judgements that are already explicitly normative.

One way to put this point is to say that, whilst normative pathological status *supervenes* on plain facts, there is no general route from a description of plain facts to pathological status. Rather, the connection is piecemeal. Having first made a judgement of mental pathology one may be able to identify aetiological factors described in non-normative terms. From these it may be possible to infer that people in relevantly similar physical states will also suffer the same illness, but this does not provide a general route to predict pathology on the basis of difference of underlying physiology. Not all physical differences correspond to pathologies.

This view of the relation between pathological status and underpinning plain facts is parallel to Donald Davidson's account of the metaphysics of mind (Davidson 1980). He suggests that whilst every individual or token mental event is a physical event—amounting to a form of monism—there is no systematic law-like connection between types of mental event and types of physical event. The same mental type might be realised by any number of different physical types. Davidson also subscribes to a version of supervenience: determining the physical facts determines the mental facts, but not vice versa. This does not licence any reduction of mental types to physical types because there is no general route from physical description to mental description, but once one has identified a type of mental event and identified how in a particular token case it is (identical with) a physical event, any other physical event of the same physical type will share the same mental type. However, there is no general route from a physical description to a mental description, which does not already presuppose identification of mental features in mental terms.

Thus, if MCI does turn out to have a predictively valid connection to Alzheimer's there is a way of resolving the question of its pathological status. It can inherit a pathological status from Alzheimer's disease as a kind of 'pre-Alzheimer's state'. Note that if this were the case, then if there were another condition that matched MCI proper as far as its symptoms were concerned but did not have this connection to Alzheimer's, it would not inherit the pathological status considered. The pathological status arrived at in this derivative way has nothing essentially to do with the experience that subjects with the symptoms of MCI suffer. MCI itself does not seem to inherit a pathological status this way. It becomes, instead, the name either for an early stage of Alzheimer's proper or, perhaps, merely a risk category for that disease.

Where does this leave the second question raised above about the pathological status of MCI? One result is that it might inherit a derivative pathological status not because there is anything essentially pathological about its symptoms, but because it transpires there is a predictively valid connection to a condition whose status is less ambiguous, even if still a matter of normative, rather than plainly descriptive, status. But, if so, there is nothing essentially pathological about the symptoms.

If instead one considers the pathological status of MCI directly, then it seems that there is no way of avoiding a difficult judgement, no short cut through consideration merely of the plain statistical facts. Instead, one has to address the question through one's preferred model of what makes a condition a disorder, disease or illness. Here, MCI remains stubbornly problematic. I will consider two models of illness or disease.

One model of the nature of illness is Fulford's failure of ordinary doing (see above). Fulford suggests that illness is an essentially evaluative notion captured by its effects on our abilities. Illness prevents us from the kind of ordinary action that is constitutive of a normal life. It is an inner block to ordinary doing. This rough outline of the analysis will do here to raise a difficulty in the case of MCI. The problem is how to apply the picture (on the assumption for the moment that the picture is correct). What should count as ordinary doing in the case of old age, given that some physiological and cognitive decline is to be expected and is accepted to be non-pathological? At what point is deviation from this ordinary decline considered to be failure? However plausible the model its underlying components will not make the facts about the pathological status of MCI more determinate.

Suppose instead that illness is explained through the notion of disorder which is in turn modelled on failures of biological function as discussed above. The problem now is that an interpretation has to be given of what the proper functions associated with ageing are. Is the usual associated physiological and cognitive decline a proper function of the human brain, or a failure of function? More plausibly, is it a contingent feature of biological traits that have other functions (perhaps active during the reproductive stages of human life), a kind of 'unintended' effect of a trait with another function? My purpose in raising this question is not to suggest an answer, but rather to highlight the fact that an answer to the parallel question about MCI would have to deliver a distinct answer if a line is to be drawn between ordinary ageing and MCI. That seems unlikely.

MCI thus appears to raise two distinct problems. First, it reminds us of the genuine distinction between the plain facts of ageing, and the pathological status of particular illnesses or diseases. This is a general feature of illness and shows the need for a particular kind of interpretative judgement. Furthermore, it presents a particular problem. The very nature of MCI appears to preclude any clear verdict about its pathological status. It may inherit that status through a connection to another, clearer condition, such as Alzheimer's. If so it is also possible that it will inherit some purely descriptive tests, which have to do with brain structure, but its pathological status has no essential connection to the signs and symptoms of MCI. On the other hand, focusing on those symptoms, there seems to be an essential ambiguity about its status.

In this section I have used mild cognitive impairment as an example of the more general problems of understanding and assessing the pathological status of mental illness. It is a study in miniature. It does, however, suggest that no purely plain or non-normative account will do either in principle or in practice.

## 5. Conclusions

Forming both an understanding of and a judgement about the debate between anti-psychiatry and descriptivist defences of psychiatry is a task for philosophy. The debate centres on a proper understanding of the nature of mental illness in particular and, it turns out, of illness in general. Whilst 'value theorists' argue that the very idea of mental illness is an essentially evaluative notion, their 'values out' opponents argue that it is a matter of the plain facts to be analysed, perhaps using the notion of biological function. A further attraction of this latter idea is that it promises to 'naturalise' illness: to place it—or at least, according to the *harmful* dysfunction analysis, a central element of it—within nature construed along the lines of merely mechanical natural science: the realm of law.

Despite the attractions of the descriptivist project, I have argued that it faces grave difficulties. A purely statistical approach cannot distinguish unusual but generally advantageous conditions—such as having a high IQ—from pathological conditions. An approach that attempts to naturalise disorder through biological or proper functions has an extra resource to address this problem. It can attempt to explain pathological behaviour in terms of a failure of biological function. Illness is thus a matter of a system not behaving as it ought to do, but, as I have argued, the extra normative quality of biological functions does not spring forth from nowhere. It is built into the selection of causal happenings from which the function is framed.

Value theorists have argued that the very idea of a biological function is an evaluative notion. Thus, they can argue that the normative character stems from values that are smuggled into the characterisation of functions. As I have argued, however, care is needed in specifying whose values are involved and precisely how. A more cautious approach is to argue that whilst functions cannot help a purely descriptive and reductionist account of illness, this need not be because of the presence of values. Rather, the pattern of explanation into which biological functions fits is the conceptually richer framework of the space of reasons, rather than the more basic realm of law. To the extent to which functions can help 'naturalise' the concept of mental illness, it is only against a broader understanding of nature.

In later chapters I will argue that psychiatry has to have a broader view of the nature of nature in other areas as well. The world contains not just what is described within mechanical natural science, the realm of law, but also aspects of the space of reasons: irreducible meanings (Chapter 4) and values (Chapters 2 and 5).

The philosophical complexities of the analysis of mental illness in general are also reflected in the analysis of particular mental illnesses. Understanding the pathological status of conditions such mild cognitive impairment calls for a judgement about the relationship of what is normal and what is pathological. Whilst models of mental illness can help in this task, ultimately there can be no avoiding a difficult judgement, which lies outside a narrow construal of empirical science.

## Chapter 2

# Values, psychiatric ethics and clinical judgement

## Plan of the chapter

1. **A toolkit for ethical reasoning in medicine and psychiatry?**
   The further challenges of psychiatric ethics
   The multiplicity of factors in psychiatric clinical judgement

2. **Judgement and the broader framework of values-based practice**
   The irreducibility of values to facts
   The subjectivity of values
   The uncodifiability of values
   Overview of the model of values that underpins values-based practice

3. **The role of judgement in the Four Principles approach to medical ethics**
   A closer look at the Four Principles approach
   Adding an account of the metaphysics of values
   Is particularism consistent with the Four Principles approach?

4. **Conclusions**

Chapter 1 examined the concept of mental illness by placing the debate about its reality in two broader contexts. One was a debate about whether illness is essentially evaluative or whether, instead, it can be given a plainly descriptive analysis. The other was a debate about how the concept of illness can be 'naturalised' or fitted into an unproblematic conception of nature. In fact, however, these are not two separate debates, but two complementary ways to view the varied disagreements between different philosophers and psychiatrists about the status of mental illness.

The debate about the nature and reality of mental illness impacts directly on psychiatric diagnosis. Because the debate is ongoing, there remains disagreement about whether diagnosis itself is value based, but it is widely agreed that treatment and management in psychiatry, like the rest of medicine, turn on values. This chapter will examine the nature of value judgements as they are more traditionally understood to impact on mental health care.

Clinical judgement in psychiatry, in so far as it is concerned with values, draws on the growing academic literature about medical ethics, but it also raises specific further issues. In this chapter I will provide a very selective overview of this difficult area, highlighting some specific complexities in the case of mental health care, but also examining how best to understand one influential approach to medical ethics generally in more detail.

Having outlined the most influential theories deployed in medical ethics, the chapter looks first at two issues that raise specific difficulties for *psychiatric* ethics: the justification for involuntary treatment and the diversity of values in mental health care. The latter has prompted the development of values-based practice initially in the context of mental health but now applied more widely. According to this view, the main aim of judgements of values in medicine should be to explore legitimate conflicts of values as the basis of balanced decision-making in particular cases, rather than aiming to arrive at a right answer through rule governed or algorithmic methods.

The second section of the chapter examines the view of values that values-based practice (VBP) presupposes. Whilst it might be thought that VBP is based on the subjectivity of value judgements, I argue that it is better to think of judgements as potentially objective, but nevertheless not algorithmic. Value judgement, like other aspects of clinical judgment, is a matter of having good, although ultimately uncodified, judgement.

The final section examines the influential Four Principles approach to medical ethics and argues that the best way to interpret this approach accords with the discussion of values-based practice. It is a form of moral 'particularism'. The chapter thus begins with specific features of psychiatric ethics, and moves in two stages to consider more general models of values and ethics, emphasising the importance for clinical judgement of a more sophisticated understanding of what good judgement in general comprises.

## 1. A toolkit for ethical reasoning in medicine and psychiatry?

Unlike many domains of philosophy, medical ethics is directly practical. One of its key roles is to frame tools to aid clinicians and other participants in clinical judgements to assess the ethical aspects of a situation. Raanan Gillon, a general practitioner and professor of medical ethics, for example, aims to demonstrate the efficacy of his favoured approach—Beauchamp and Childress' Four Principles approach—by showing how it can simplify a range of factors that might otherwise have to be assessed individually. In a paper called 'Ethics needs principles—four can encompass the rest—and respect for autonomy should be "first among equals"', Gillon considers another ethicist's analysis of the merits of a free market in human organs, and draws from it the following daunting list of the relevant considerations:

- people's rights and claims;
- different sorts of interests and their relative strength;
- human wellbeing;
- loss of life;
- what would be good or bad for people;
- democratic acceptance;
- consultation;
- sensitive moments;
- benefits and harms;
- grief and distress;
- an obligation to make sacrifices for the community;
- an entitlement of the community to deny autonomy and even to violate bodily integrity in the public interest;
- the system of justice;
- public safety;
- public policy considerations;
- danger;
- civil liberties;
- individual autonomy;
- saving and protecting the lives and liberties of citizens (Gillon 2003: 308).

He goes on to say: 'my hypothesis entails that all of them can be explained and justified by one or some combination of the four principles' (Gillon 2003: 308). Thus, one role for a philosophical theory of medical ethics—a theory of normative ethics, of how one ought to act—is to codify and rank competing factors to guide judgement.

Perhaps the best known approaches to medical ethics are three general moral philosophy perspectives—consequentialism, deontology and virtue ethics—and one specifically medical ethical (and deontological) approach: the Four Principles.

Very briefly they are as follows.

## Consequentialism

As its name suggests, this is the view that the moral value of an ethical judgement or action depends only on whether it has good consequences. That simple characterisation hides an immediate further complexity. How should the good consequences be characterised? If the aim is to explain moral judgements in other terms—to reduce moral to non-moral concepts—then the consequences might be, for example, defined in terms of human happiness. Thus, moral judgement would be explained as that which leads to happy consequences, morally good, thus being explained using a non-moral concept of happiness. Of course, like any reductionist definition, it is open to question whether the concept of moral good can be explained using non-moral concepts. A more modest non-reductive form of consequentialism, by contrast, might instead help itself only to a morally rich notion of 'good consequences' or morally good consequences. This would not attempt to shed light on what is meant by 'morality' from the outside, but might still help to emphasise that what matters are the effects of, rather than the motives for, moral actions.

The most famous instance of a consequentialist approach is JS Mill's Utilitarianism, which Mill summarises as follows:

> The creed which accepts as the foundation of morals, Utility, or the Greatest Happiness Principle, holds that actions are right in proportion as they tend to promote happiness, wrong as they tend to produce the reverse of happiness. By happiness is intended pleasure, and the absence of pain; by unhappiness, pain, and the privation of pleasure. To give a clear view of the moral standard set up by the theory, much more requires to be said; in particular, what things it includes in the ideas of pain and pleasure; and to what extent this is left an open question. But these supplementary explanations do not affect the theory of life on which this theory of morality is grounded - namely, that pleasure, and freedom from pain, are the only things desirable as ends; and that all desirable things (which are as numerous in the utilitarian as in any other scheme) are desirable either for the pleasure inherent in themselves, or as means to the promotion of pleasure and the prevention of pain. (Mill 1979: 7)

Utilitarianism lies at the heart of the assessment of healthcare in terms of the QALY or Quality Adjusted Life Year, which forms the basis of quasi-economic assessment of competing claims for resources. The basic idea is that a year of life enjoyed with full health is given a numerical value of one. A less than fully healthy year of life scores less on a scale, which reflects the experienced quality. The value of medical care can then be assessed by predicting the outcome expressed in QALY relative to the economic cost. (In 2004, the chief executive of NICE in the UK reported to a seminar at the University of Warwick that, as a matter of fact, decisions recently made by NICE had tended to favour treatments costing less than £30,000 per QALY.)

A central challenge for consequentialists is to reconcile the idea that the moral value of an action depends upon a kind of calculus of outcomes with our everyday ignorance of the longer term consequences of our actions. Another problem is that a utilitarian calculation may threaten individual rights if collective happiness or good sufficiently outweighs—according to consequentialist or utilitarian calculation—individual suffering. However, the idea that individual rights can be so outweighed may not accord with antecedent intuitions about morality.

## Deontology

On this approach, the moral value of an action is independent of the action's actual consequences but depends instead on one or more general duties to act. Particular kinds of action are simply precluded or, contrastingly, demanded by general principles. The challenge for its supporters is thus to articulate a consistent set of principles or general duties that capture morally correct action and to explain their origin. Some duties, such as the Hippocratic injunction to do no harm, are widely and deeply held, but as I will explain below, can conflict with other equally deeply held principles to do patients good.

The most famous form of deontological theory is Kantian ethics, which centres on a single high level 'categorical imperative' or principle:

♦ Act only according to that maxim by which you can at the same time will that it should become a universal law.

This flows from Kant's argument that the key feature of morality is that moral guidance must be capable of application in any possible set of circumstances. Generality is of the essence of morality, on this view.

However, even this formal constraint has content because some maxims would be self-stultifying if generalised. Consider the putative maxim that it is permissible to steal. If this were generalised, it would undermine the possibility of owning property in general, but if so, stealing would not, after all, be possible.

In addition to ruling out some actions because a maxim derived from it could not be generalised without contradiction, the first formulation of the categorical imperative also gives rise to more specific advice. Kant's view of morality is based on a highly rationalist view. A moral agent should want to do what is good not for any subjective reasons—such as hypothetical imperatives that if one wants such and such an end then one should adopt such and such an means—but for an absolutely or categorically compelling end. Thus, free will is a basic precondition of moral action, albeit a will to be governed by absolute principles and, if it is to be universalised, it would contradict the categorical imperative as set out above to claim that a person is merely a means to some other end, rather than always an end in his or her self. Hence, Kant gives a further derivation of the first imperative:

♦ Act in such a way that you always treat humanity, whether in your own person or in the person of any other, never simply as a means, but always at the same time as an end.

The main challenge to a Kantian version of deontology is to show how all the intuitively morally compelling principles can be derived from the formal requirement for universality. The challenge for any version of deontology that accepts a basic plurality of principles is to explain away the problem that they may conflict in particular circumstances (see below).

## Virtue ethics

On this approach, the moral value of ethical judgement depends on the character of a moral subject. The fullest original statement was Aristotle's *Nicomachean Ethics* (Aristotle 2000). The central practical aim of virtue ethics is the development of a moral character. Thus, one of the Aristotle's key tasks is to offer an account of the sort of characteristics a virtuous person has (and from which the value of ethical judgements derives). The ultimate aim of virtue ethics is *eudaemonia*, meaning flourishing. Thus success in ethical judgements is underpinned by a conception of a good, happy and fulfilling life. It is a matter of debate whether the concept of a good life is always morally charged or whether, by contrast, some kind of reduction of moral properties to some non-moral form of the good life is intended.

## The Four Principles

The Four Principles approach is a deontological approach set out at length by Tom Beauchamp and James Childress in their *Principles of Biomedical Ethics* (Beauchamp and Childress 2001). In it, the authors set out four general principles to guide medical ethical reasoning:

- *Autonomy:* The patient or user's perspective is fundamental and informed consent to treatment is thus a key derivative ethical aim.
- *Beneficence:* The good of the patient is a key aim.
- *Non-maleficence:* Harm should be avoided where possible.
- *Justice:* Benefits, risks and costs should be distributed fairly. Subjects in similar positions should be treated in a similar manner.

These four principles are supposed to capture medical ethical reasoning. They do not derive from any single higher principle. As I will explain further towards the end of this chapter, they need both 'balancing' and further 'specification' when applied to particular situations because the principles can conflict. For example, beneficence and non-maleficence are in tension in both surgery and drug treatment. In psychiatry, in particular, autonomy and beneficence are in tension in the case of involuntary treatment.

Even a brief summary of these four distinct general approaches reveals the conceptual and practical difficulties of medical ethics (and there are many other approaches including narrative ethics and casuistry). First, the rival ethical models or theories need to be fully articulated. Secondly, because they can give different results, a justified choice has to be made about which to follow. A consequentialist or utilitarian approach might suggest that the consequences of Robin Hood's actions are sufficiently good to justify stealing from the rich. A deontological approach might insist that stealing is always, as a matter of principle, wrong. Thirdly, the 'data'—the full details of clinical situations—have to be interpreted and related to favoured medical ethical theories. Fourthly, a judgement has to be derived from the favoured theory as applied to the case at hand. At each of these stages, there can be reasonable disagreement between different parties. Such judgements lack reliability in the medical sense.

## The further challenges of psychiatric ethics

Whatever the practical and conceptual difficulties of medical ethics in general, psychiatric ethics reflects further complexities in mental health care. These can be divided into two areas:

- difficulties raised by core features of mental health care;
- difficulties raised by the multiplicity of values implicitly or explicitly in play in mental health care.

I will take these in turn in this and the next subsection.

Mental health care is unique in medicine in that it is an area where fully conscious adult patients of normal intelligence can be treated against their will. Furthermore, the legitimacy of such treatment turns on an essential, albeit contested, aspect of mental illness. It is of the very nature of some mental illnesses that sufferers should be treated despite their objections. That, of course, is to put the case from the perspective of an opponent of antipsychiatry. According to a follower of Szasz (see Chapter 1) matters look very different. Because there is no such thing as mental illness—that is when construed as both a deviation from evaluative norms, but also medically treatable—then there is no excuse for the detention and treatment of supposed sufferers (sufferers at worst of moral or other life problems). The debate about the reality of mental illness thus impacts directly on the ethical issue of compulsory treatment.

Paul Chodoff, a professor of psychiatry and prolific author on psychiatric ethics, writing in 1984, sets out the conflict of views on this central aspect of mental health care as follows:

> I have ... noted ... that (as happens whenever differing opinions are held with emotional intensity) a complex matter has become polarized into blacks and whites. On the one hand there are those who regret the necessity for involuntary hospitalization but regard it as an essential last resort enabling the care and treatment of a small proportion of patients whose severe mental illnesses substantially interfere with their

capacity to accept such treatment voluntarily. This is the medical model approach and I count myself among its adherents along with, I believe, a majority of psychiatrists and some lawyers as well. The contrary position is maintained in varying degrees by a smaller articulate segment of the psychiatric profession and by a number of lawyers ... This is the civil liberties approach. Those who hold it have in common the conviction that the psychiatric hospitalization of a person against his or her will is a dangerous assault on individual freedom. The members of this group, however, are by no means monolithic in the intensity with which they oppose involuntary hospitalization. Some of them support Szaszian absolutism. They regard forced hospitalization of anyone for the sake of his mental health as anathema; there are no circumstances under which it can be justified. Another and currently more influential civil liberties position is to accept forced hospitalization under certain circumstances but only in the most gingerly fashion and when hedged about with rigid restrictions. (Chodoff 1984: 384)

Chodoff's summary reflects in part the more general rise of the civil liberties movement and the increasing stress on autonomy in medicine. That emphasis has grown with the rise of the view as patient as consumer, especially with growing awareness of the costs of medical care and the issue of who ultimately pays those costs. Nevertheless, it is neither a recent nor a local phenomenon:

A basic tenet of medical ethics is that people whose body is to be interfered with, be it for therapeutic and/or research purposes, ought to be fully informed about the intended procedure prior to expressing their uncoerced, explicit and revocable acceptance to participate. This interactive process was first proclaimed for research protocols in 1933, only to be shamelessly disregarded and violated by the German Nazi dictatorship. International recognition of the fundamental right to informed consent was initially obtained through the Declaration of Nuremberg (1947) and ratified by the successive Declarations of Helsinki (1964–2000) and others, extending it to patients' involvement in the institution, omission or suspension of medical treatment that directly concerns them. (Kottow 2004: 565)

Thus, one key medical and moral value is the right of a subject to agree to, or refuse, treatment. In mental health care, however, this value is not sacrosanct and can be outweighed by concern for the subject's health. In the terms of Beauchamp and Childress' Four Principles approach, the heart of the challenge psychiatry presents is a conflict between autonomy and beneficence. This conflict runs very deep and, in practice, generally leads to a kind of compromise between what Chodoff calls a medical model approach and a moderate version of civil liberties. As Bill Fulford observes:

Decisions about compulsory treatment, although essentially medical decisions, and life-and-death decisions at that, are none the less firmly among those which society is unwilling to leave solely to doctors alone. (Fulford 1989: 189)

What underpins this compromise? How can the conflict between autonomy and beneficence, and the reason why, in mental health care, autonomy can be outweighed, be best understood? Rather than starting with the more difficult case of the justification of involuntary treatment I will start with the easier inverse case of why the conditions that have to be met for informed consent may not be met in the case of mental illness. (Of course, the fact that someone cannot give informed consent does not itself justify their involuntary treatment.)

In a useful short summary paper, two South African psychiatrists summarise some of these conditions:

> Notwithstanding standard conditions such as information, trust, and lack of coercion, we shall confine the consideration of the conditions necessary for informed consent to those that typically cannot be met owing to mental disorder. Thus, they are presented not as sufficient conditions, but each of them being necessary. They are:
>
> I.   a mental disorder should not prevent a patient from *understanding* what s/he consents to;
>
> II.  a mental disorder should not prevent a patient from *choosing* decisively for/against the intervention;
>
> III. a mental disorder should not prevent a patient from *communicating* his/her consent (presuming that at least reasonable steps have been taken to understand the patient's communication if present at all), and
>
> IV.  a mental disorder should not prevent a patient from *accepting* the need for a medical intervention. (Van Staden and Kruger 2006: 41)

These conditions, however, can present practical difficulties in the case of mental illness where subjects lack insight into their illness. Such a lack of insight may be compatible with satisfaction of the first three conditions, but not the fourth:

> The problem is that mental disorder prevents some patients from accepting that they need a medical intervention. We see this particularly in patients suffering from psychotic illnesses, such as schizophrenia. They may understand the treatment proposed, but still decline or refuse it because, in their judgment, they are not ill or do not need treatment for their difficulties. For example, a patient suffering from psychotic illness may assert adamantly: I understand that you think I am ill, I understand your proposed treatment and potential consequences of my taking or my not taking the treatment, but I am *not* ill, or: I know I am ill, I understand the proposed nature and purposes of the treatment, but I don't need treatment for it, because my illness will disappear in the near future when I will be God. Such impaired judgment in patients suffering from psychotic illnesses is inherent to their illness. We clinicians commonly refer to this kind of judgment about their state of health as a lack of insight into their condition. (Van Staden and Kruger 2006: 42)

The problem at the heart of these necessary conditions is one of insight or its lack. If a subject lacks insight into their condition then they cannot offer informed consent:

> However, in the case of a patient who cannot accept that an intervention is warranted or necessary, *owing to a mental disorder*, such a patient's choice is not autonomous

because it is determined by the mental disorder. This also means that even if such a patient were to agree to an intervention, it would be farfetched to attest that s/he actually gave informed consent. (Van Staden and Kruger 2006: 42)

To return to the more contentious, though reciprocal issue of compulsory treatment, it might seem that such treatment can be justified by a lack of insight, but what kind of lack of insight justifies such treatment and why?

Fulford, for example, notes that lack of insight comes in different kinds. He gives an example, borrowed from the psychiatrist Aubrey Lewis, of a doctor with acromegaly (a hormonal disorder involving excess growth hormone) who 'for twenty years failed to perceive his own progressive facial disfigurement' (Fulford 1989: 195). That doctor clearly lacked insight into his condition. Indeed, many people refuse to believe severe and unfortunate diagnoses through a kind of wishful thinking.

However, such lack of insight is not in itself a justification for compulsory treatment. It is only a lack of insight in a form which is characteristic of some forms of mental illness, notably functional psychotic mental illness characterized by the presence of delusions, that is the paradigm for justifying compulsory treatment. The ethical challenge here is thus to unpack the reason why certain kinds of lack of insight justify compulsory treatment, whilst others do not. Fulford himself aims to shed light on this by connecting the issue of compulsory treatment to the way in which psychotic loss of insight emerges as a central kind of psychopathology within his agency-based analysis of illness outlined in Chapter 1, as (or as being derived from) a particular kind of 'failure of ordinary doing'. Conventional function-based accounts, as Fulford shows, actually marginalize psychotic loss of insight (Aubrey Lewis famously disowned it!), but on Fulford's account:

> [T]he experience of illness in general is to be interpreted in terms of disturbance in the machinery of action. Hence, on this model, the variety especially of mental illness experiences (i.e. of psychopathology) can be interpreted as disturbances of different kinds and in different parts of this machinery. There is good evidence, as with values, that we draw on notions of agency even in our scientific classifications of mental disorder. Reasons, however, have a central place in this machinery. Sensation, movement, volition, memory, perception, etc. are all executive—they are all necessary to the *carrying out* of an action. But reasons *define the action itself* ... If, therefore, reasons (of this reasons-for-action kind), are a central rather than merely executive component of action, psychotic illness as a *disturbance* of reasons-for-action, emerges quite naturally in an action-failure account of psychopathology, as the central kind of mental illness. (Fulford 1999a: 184)

In other words, by analysing illness in terms of failure of action, Fulford's model suggests that differences between kinds of illness are constituted by different kinds of failure of action. In most cases, including all cases of physical illness, the failure is a failure of one kind or another to execute an intact act. In paradigmatically psychotic forms of mental illness, however, the failure is more fundamental. It concerns a failure or defect of what Aristotle first called 'reasons for actions', the reasons, that is, by which the very act itself is defined.

It is worth looking at this point in a little more detail, since it is here that there is a crucial break between Fulford's agency-based account of the subject's experience of illness with, as I will argue, its implicit links to the uncodifiability of judgement, and more traditional function-based accounts of disease and disorder. Thus, within any function-based accounts, defects of reasoning are treated as defects of particular cognitive functions, but the particular cognitive functions of people with delusions—their memory, intelligence and so forth—are intact, notably in the paradigmatic monosymptomatic delusional disorders. Fulford's agency-based account, by contrast, connects the relevant kind of defect of reasoning directly with the reasons that, as whole persons, actually define our actions as our own. Fulford's arguments in support of this connection are rather technical, but they are based on the close phenomenological parallels between reasons (as in 'reasons for action') and the clinical psychopathology of delusions. Granted these phenomenological parallels, therefore, and the general framework of an agency-based account of the experience of illness, physical as well as mental, the special ethical status of psychotic loss of insight falls out of the theory quite naturally, for this kind of insight represents a *constitutive*, rather than merely executive, failure of action.

The next stage of the argument aims to connect this analysis of a fundamental kind of mental illness to the justification for compulsory treatment. Why should such a deep failure within a subject's reasons for action justify compulsory treatment? Fulford suggests that light can be shed on this by noting how this same fundamental kind of mental illness, involving psychotic loss of insight, can serve to *excuse* actions alongside more everyday excuses: accident, mistake and impaired consciousness. Here, calling his own action-theoretic approach the 'reverse-view' (because it starts with the experience of illness of subjects rather than underlying medical explanations), Fulford argues:

> [I]n the case of mental illness as an excuse, it is more immediately clear why a reverse-view analysis gives the right result, allowing, where a conventional-view analysis fails to allow, mental illness the moral properties it (intuitively) has. For the factor common to each of the standard excuses—accident, mistake, impaired consciousness—is lack of intent. And it is just this that is implied by a reverse-view analysis of 'psychosis'. All non-psychotic illnesses, analysed in reverse-view terms, involve... instrumental failures of 'ordinary' doing, difficulties in doing what one intends to do. And difficulties of this sort often mitigate and, if very severe, may even excuse. But in the case of psychotic illness, the failure of 'ordinary' doing implied by a reverse-view analysis is a

failure in the very specification of what is done. The psychotic, therefore... lacks intent... [H]e is thus in the same position as others who lack intent in that he is not responsible for what he does, and, hence, excused. Responsibility, however, is closely linked with rights... [G]ranted this link, if a reverse-view account of 'psychosis' explains so straightforwardly why the psychotic is not responsible for what he does, then this is indeed a clear indication that a reverse-view account should also be capable of explaining that most obscure of moral phenomena, the loss of rights necessary to the justification of compulsory psychiatric treatment. (Fulford 1989: 242–3)

The idea here is that the more basic notion that lack of intent excuses an action can be connected through two links to the problem of justifying compulsory treatment. First, psychotic illness, in which a subject lacks insight into his or her condition, undermines the subject's capacity to form reasons (in the relevant sense, as above) and thus connects to defective intent. Secondly, a subject whose purported actions can be excused by defective intent (which may undermine their status *as* actions: a slip is not an action) is also by that fact the kind of subject whose autonomy can justifiably be overridden.

As Fulford spells out, there is of course a sense in which people with psychotic loss of insight clearly do form intentions, just as there is a sense in which they clearly do have reasons for their actions. The point is rather that, to the extent that their actions reflect psychotic loss of insight, their reasons are defective, in whatever (as yet to be determined) way delusional reasoning is defective. Defective reasons for action imply defective intentions, and, hence, excuse.

This general approach promises to shed light on the key justification for compulsory treatment. There are, however, still some questions remaining. Do all cases that merit compulsory treatment involve defective intent? Why precisely does such a defect justify treatment? What exactly is the connection between the possibility of excusing purported actions because of some failure of intent and overriding the agent's remaining autonomy? What precisely comprises a relevant defect of intent? Is it right to say that there is a lack of intent, a failure within the specification of intention or an impaired intention or what? Nevertheless, it suggests that psychiatry carries with it quite specific medical ethical complexities which flow from the fact that it centres on disorders of human agency.

## The multiplicity of factors in psychiatric clinical judgement

The second additional complexity for psychiatric, rather than more generically medical, ethics concerns the multiplicity of factors in play which are either values themselves or directly relevant to value judgements.

Recall the analysis developed by Bill Fulford and outlined in Chapter 1. According to Fulford, mental illness shares with physical illness an essentially evaluative nature. There is no prospect for a purely descriptive or 'values out' account of illness through, for example, the notion of failure of biological function. There is, however, a greater appearance of values in mental health care because of a feature of the relation of values and factual criteria. Where values are agreed, descriptive criteria can go proxy for them. That is the case in much physical medicine, but it is not so in mental health care and, consequently, the differing values are more apparent here.

One broad way to think of this difference is to note the greater extent to which rival conceptions of human flourishing (or *eudaemonia*) are implicated in mental health care by contrast with, for example, cardiology. There is widespread agreement about the usefulness for more or less any kind of human flourishing of a well functioning heart. Furthermore, within the limits of public understanding of biology, there is widespread lay agreement about what that good functioning comprises (even if this is limited to 'whatever is necessary for enabling an active life'). By contrast, in conditions as diverse as anorexia, personality disorder and depression there can be marked differences in the assessment—between, but not only between, subject and clinician—of what *eudaemonia* might properly be said to involve. For that reason, attention to the possibility of diverse values is all the more practically important.

In addition to diversity of the values which are either—according to value-theorists—partly constitutive of mental illness or—for descriptivists—at least closely associated with their treatment, there are also other factors that impact on values. These include key notions that cannot be taken for granted in mental illness. They include capacity, autonomy, rationality, intention, personal identity and so forth. In each case, a notion that might be taken for granted and, thus, perhaps not even explicitly considered in physical medicine has to be explicitly investigated in mental health care.

Given this complexity and drawing on his analysis of mental illness, Bill Fulford has proposed some principles to guide what he calls values-based practice drawn originally from consideration of mental health care, but now applied to medicine more generally. The principles are explicitly intended to complement evidence-based medicine (EBM) in framing clinical judgements. However, unlike EBM, the principles that guide value judgements are not aimed at algorithmically determining a right answer, but rather exploring legitimate differences of view.

In the next section I will outline those principles and consider the model of values on which the principles are based. This will move the chapter's discussion from the values and ethics of mental health specifically to a broader context and the very idea of values in play. The final section will examine in more detail the application of the Four Principles approach in medical ethical judgement drawing on the discussion to come of values-based practice to argue for the importance of non-algorithmic and uncodifiable one-off judgements in the face of complex situations.

## 2. Judgement and the broader framework of values-based practice

'Values-based practice' (VBP) has been developed recently in the UK to guide clinical judgements in mental health care and also more broadly. VBP is the practical counterpart of the analysis of values in medicine proposed by Bill Fulford and outlined in Chapter 1. The main emphasis in VBP is that clinical decision making, to the extent that it involves values, is not sufficiently guided by a framework of ethical rules and regulation, important as such a framework is, but depends also on learnable clinical skills to respond in a balanced way to a far broader range of diverse values. Values-based practice thus shifts the emphasis in clinical decision-making from 'right outcomes', defined by ethical rules and regulation, to 'good process'. It provides a skills-based approach to balanced decision-making where, as is often particularly the case in mental health, complex and conflicting values are in play.

A number of the key elements of the good process of values-based practice have been summarised by Fulford in the form of ten principles, as set out below. As will be seen, four key areas of clinical skill (awareness, knowledge, reasoning and communication) are defined by principles 6–9, but the good process of values-based practice also depends on recognising the close interdependence of values and evidence (principles 1–3), on patient-centred and multidisciplinary service delivery (principles 4 and 5, respectively) and, perhaps most important of all, on a partnership approach to clinical decision-making in which the locus of control shifts from outside experts (including lawyer and ethicists) to the particular individuals directly concerned in a given decision.

## Ten principles of values-based practice
(From Fulford 2004: 205–34)

1: All decisions stand on two feet, on values as well as on facts, including decisions about diagnosis (the "two feet" principle)

2: We tend to notice values only when they are diverse or conflicting and hence are likely to be problematic (the "squeaky wheel" principle)

**Ten principles of values-based practice** (From Fulford 2004: 205–34) *(continued)*

3: Scientific progress, in opening up choices, is increasingly bringing the full diversity of human values into play in all areas of healthcare (the "science driven" principle)

4: VBP's "first call" for information is the perspective of the patient or patient group concerned in a given decision (the "patient-perspective" principle)

5: In VBP, conflicts of values are resolved primarily, not by reference to a rule prescribing a "right" outcome, but by processes designed to support a balance of legitimately different perspectives (the "multi-perspective" principle)

6: Careful attention to language use in a given context is one of a range of powerful methods for raising awareness of values (the "values-blindness" principle)

7: A rich resource of both empirical and philosophical methods is available for improving our knowledge of other people's values (the "values-myopia" principle)

8: Ethical reasoning is employed in VBP primarily to explore differences of values, not, as in quasi-legal bioethics, to determine "what is right" (the "space of values" principle)

9: In VBP, communication skills have a substantive rather than (as in quasi-legal ethics) a merely executive role in clinical decision-making (the "how it's done" principle)

10: VBP, although involving a partnership with ethicists and lawyers (equivalent to the partnership with scientists and statisticians in EBM), puts decision-making back where it belongs, with users and providers at the clinical coal-face (the "who decides" principle)

In the UK, these principles or pointers to balanced decision-making in mental health practice have been increasingly influential in a number of recent mental health care initiatives. One very concrete instance is a training manual, published by the Sainsbury Centre for Mental Health, called *Whose values? A workbook for values-based practice in mental health care* (Woodbridge and Fulford 2004). That workbook in turn has been the basis for a number of policy, training and service development initiatives rolled out through the UK government's Department of Health and, internationally, particularly through the World Psychiatric Association. My aim here, however, is not to look to those practical applications, but to explore the underlying philosophical model of values that best fits this approach.

For this aim, three of these principles—2, 5 and 8—are particularly important. They bring out the characteristic logic of values. We notice values only when they are diverse because, as described in Chapter 1, when they are agreed they can become submerged beneath factual criteria. However, when there is disagreement about values, there is no decision procedure to lead all parties to agreement. Furthermore, in so far as principles can be used, they do not serve the role set out for them in a principles-driven account of medical ethics. What, precisely, do these claims presuppose about the nature of values?

I will consider three claims:

- ◆ the irreducibility of values to facts;
- ◆ the subjectivity of values; and
- ◆ the uncodifiability of values.

## The irreducibility of values to facts

Fulford's analysis requires a distinction between facts and values (strictly, description and evaluation). The account he gives of the dependence of factual criteria for disease concepts, for example, on underlying values requires a distinction between them. If the values apparently implicit in illness could be reduced in some way to facts then the position would collapse into the purely factual view of illness put forward by biologically-minded opponents of anti-psychiatry whom Fulford criticises.

There is no knock-down argument for the 'values in' view of mental illness. Nevertheless, as outlined in Chapter 1, two kinds of consideration support it. First, as Fulford in particular has argued, ordinary linguistic uses of all the medical concepts—disorder, disease, illness, and so forth—suggest a *prima facie* connection to values. To repeat, this can be disguised if there is sufficient agreement about the values involved to permit a kind of factual shorthand. Remember from Chapter 1 that where the factual criteria for the value judgments expressed by a given value term are widely shared or agreed upon, these factual criteria may come to be strongly associated with the use of that value term. In short, a value term, in these circumstances, may come to look like a factual term. However, that does not undermine the fundamental priority of the value-laden concept of illness over whatever factual criteria can contingently be used to label particular diseases and disorders.

Secondly, the opposing programme aiming to show how apparent values can in fact be reduced to underlying facts faces grave difficulties. The most promising approach is to reduce illness or disease or disorder to dysfunction and give a purely descriptive account of natural function, but there are two kinds of objections to this (outlined in Chapter 1). First, it is by no means clear that selecting particular functional explanations from the full and complex history of biological happenings is just a matter of description (Fulford 1999a,b; Thornton 2000). Secondly, even if that were possible, the connection between illness and failure of function is not straightforward (Cooper 2002).

A conceptual distinction between values and facts also fits with a broader distinction between normative and non-normative concepts that will be discussed and defended in Chapters 3 and 4. The distinction, introduced in Chapter 1, between the 'space of reasons' and the 'realm of law' will play an important role in those later chapters to contrast the normativity of meaning and mental content, and the norm-free plain facts that make up underlying neurology. Thus, whilst not implied by those later chapters, a distinction between values and facts here better fits the overall anti-reductionist view of psychiatry that will emerge. (There have also been arguments put forward by the philosophers Hilary Putnam and John Searle against a separation of fact and value but see Chapter 1 for criticism of these. In Putnam's terms, all that is required is a distinction rather than a dichotomy of fact and value.)

On the assumption, therefore, that values are distinct from and irreducible to facts, what else about them is presupposed by VBP?

## The subjectivity of values

One possibility is the claim that values are subjective. This fits with and helps explain the irreducibility thesis. If values are subjective then they belong to a different ontological kind from facts and hence cannot be reduced to them. There are a number of different ways in which this basic claim can be articulated within a broader theory of values, many deriving from one kind of interpretation of the work of the Scottish philosopher David Hume.

The starting point for such neo-Humeanism is that values are not part of the fabric of the world but are instead projected onto it as a result of the inner sentiments we feel. Whilst we may say that an action is good this is not because the action has a real property of goodness. Rather, we feel good about the action—we say 'hooray!' to it—and then project that inner feeling onto the action, mistakenly taking the feeling to be bound up in the action itself. That general approach can be incorporated within a more precise philosophical theory of values in a number of different ways.

According to one view, all value judgements are strictly false because there are no values 'out there' although just such a picture of values is presupposed by everyday value judgements (Mackie 1977). A less revisionary view concedes that value judgements cannot be true or false in the same objective way as other empirical judgements but nevertheless attempts to define a kind of 'as if' truth for them. The philosopher Simon Blackburn calls this position 'quasi-realism' (Blackburn 2000). Such details, however, do not matter here. The fundamental shared assumption of neo-Humeanism is that values do not form part of the fabric of the world and that explains the distinction between facts and values. Values are irreducible to facts because the former are subjective and the latter are objective.

The claim that values are subjective would also fit a claim from the framework of values-based practice set out above. Within a VBP approach, even ethical reasoning (not just reasoning about personal values and preferences) aims to *explore* differences of values, rather than, as in quasi-legal bioethics, to determine what is right. A subjective view undermines the possibility of a definitive end point and hence puts the emphasis on the exploratory processes instead.

Despite the attractions of the view that values are subjective, it has two kinds of disadvantage. The first is practical. Whilst some value judgements appear to be subjective, others do not. It is plausible, for example, to take preferences about the best pizza topping to answer to nothing objective in the world, but the moral repulsion felt by most people over the murders committed by the UK general practitioner Harold Shipman suggests, *prima facie*, a deeper genuine disagreement. It is not merely that Shipman had a legitimately different preference when it came to the relation between general practice and murder of the elderly.

A further practical point concerns the requirement—hinted at in principles 5 and 8 of VBP—to attempt to explore and balance differing values. What value does this requirement have? It does not seem to be, nor logically could it be, merely a subjective preference. In order that the approach to value judgements summarised in these principles is to have significant value itself, then this principle had better have more than a subjective status. If so, then at least some value judgements cannot be subjective.

The second is a philosophical point. The theory that value judgements are based on projections of inner sentiments requires a separation of complex judgement into two factors: real and objective features of the world, on the one hand, which prompt inner sentiments and attitudes, on the other. Moral and other evaluative reactions, on which moral and value judgements are based, are explained by the interplay of these two factors. The challenge for the kind of subjectivism under consideration is to give a non-question-begging account of the two factors. Neither seems to be an unproblematic task.

Take the case of the attitude or inner sentiment. The question is how this can be independently characterised. The philosopher John McDowell considers the analogous case of giving a projective account of judgements about what is funny, based on our responses:

> But what exactly is it that we are to conceive as projected on to the world so as to give rise to our idea that things are funny? "An inclination to laugh" is not a satisfactory answer; projecting an inclination to laugh would not necessarily yield an apparent

instance of the comic, since laughter can signal, for instance, embarrassment just as well as amusement. Perhaps the right response cannot be identified except as amusement; and perhaps amusement cannot be understood except as finding something comic ... But if it is correct, there is a serious question whether we can really *explain* the idea of something's being comic as a *projection* of that response ... [as] there is no self-contained prior fact of our subjective lives that could enter into a projective account of the relevant way of thinking ... No doubt the propensity to laugh is in some sense a self-contained prior psychological fact. But differentiating some exercises of that unspecific propensity as cases of *amusement* is something we have to learn ... and this learning is indistinguishable from coming to find some things comic. (McDowell 1998b: 158)

The implication of the example is this. If moral and other evaluative reactions are to be *explained* as the projection onto the world of sentiments it had better be possible to characterise those sentiments other than in terms of reactions to worldly features. In the case of comedy, this seems impossible. Moral reactions seem even harder to characterise in terms independent of reactions to worldly, but moral features.

It is worth mentioning a complementary difficulty. The inner sentiment is supposed to be prompted by genuine, but value-free, features of the external world. This raises the question: what kind of pattern is there, expressible in value-free terms, which prompts the inner sentiments. What, for example, do all cruel actions have in common except for being cruel? Again, a two-factor explanation needs to analyse a moral reaction into two independent factors: a genuine, but value-free pattern in the outer world and inner sentiments also characterised other than as a reaction to evaluative features of the world, but neither factor seems to be describable independently of the other.

Subjectivism about values cannot be defeated either by pointing out its *prima facie* implausibility or even pointing out its deeper explanatory difficulties. However, these factors do suggest that suspicion about realism about values may well be misplaced. There remain some open questions. The argument derived from McDowell suggests that a neo-Humean projectivist analysis of value judgements of even what is comic fails, but is it really true that all value judgements have equal status and are equally objective? Why is it that some judgements, such as judgements of mere preference (about pizza toppings), seem to be merely subjective. I will, however, leave those questions open here drawing the conclusion merely that there is reason to be suspicious of a universally subjective account of value judgements and turn instead to a different approach to values that could also underpin values-based practice.

## The uncodifiability of values

Rather than claiming that values are subjective, however, it is possible to make a distinct claim and still preserve much of the framework for value judgements summarised above. This is the claim that value judgements cannot be codified; they cannot be exhaustively summarised by, or in, principles.

Two kinds of consideration support this claim. One is simply appearance. To an unprejudiced eye, it should be apparent that judgements about conflicting values are made in the absence of a general theory. This point is best made by looking to a non-medical and comparatively trivial example because it is easier to consider matters where the stakes are low. Consider, for example, how one might make choices in a pizzeria. One may have in mind some general maxims such as:

♦ a spicy pizza is best accompanied by a fruity red wine like Zinfandel;

♦ there is no point in eating a mozzarella garlic bread and also pizza at the same meal;

♦ any pizza with egg on it should be treated with suspicion;

♦ all unbaked cheesecakes are an abomination;

♦ one should never spend more than £50 for two at a pizzeria.
  On any particular visit, one might have some particular initial desires:

♦ to have a glass of Sauvignon Blanc;

♦ to eat a pizza with capers;

♦ to start with a cheesy garlic bread;

♦ to eat cheesecake;

♦ to have truffle and so on.

These particular desires and more general maxims then have to be balanced. Perhaps the only pizza with capers also has egg; there is no wine available by the glass, but a bottle of white and a bottle of fruity red will threaten the budget; the waiter is not sure whether the cheesecake is baked, and so on. Steering a steady course through these inter-related factors is part of the small scale drama of everyday value judgements. Ultimately, however, whilst some general principles may help, they run out. (A possible exception to this is expressed in the anecdote that the philosopher Ludwig Wittgenstein did not mind what he ate as long as it was always the same.)

In the trivial example just sketched, there is only one relevant party to the decision and, aside from financial considerations, the values are all gastronomic. Nevertheless, the judgement about what to order cannot be codified as an argument. In medicine in general and in psychiatry in particular, matters are much more complex. There are usually a number of relevant parties to a clinical judgement and a range of different kinds of values in play, from simple preferences to deeply held moral values. Thus, to an unprejudiced eye, it should be apparent that it is unlikely that such judgements could be codified.

Despite those appearances, however, it is tempting to think that if a judgement is not merely an act of arbitrary picking but is instead rationally guided by factors then it *must* be guided by a principle. The second consideration, therefore, is an argument to undermine this prejudice about the nature of rationality. It is drawn from the later work of Ludwig Wittgenstein (1889–1951), the Cambridge-based Austrian philosopher. This is the first of three places in this book in which Wittgenstein's discussion of rule following plays a role (the others are in the discussion of understanding meaning in Chapter 4 and the role of tacit knowledge in clinical judgement in Chapter 6). For now a brief summary will suffice (see Chapter 6 for the fullest presentation).

To anticipate a little, an important general point that the work of Wittgenstein and his interpreters brings out is that the failure of full codification is not just a feature of value judgements, but all judgements, including those in science and mathematics. For some judgements including, paradigmatically, mathematical judgements, correctness can be summarised in a principle or principles, but correctly following the codification ultimately depends, not on a further principle, but on a basic judgement of what the most natural continuation is. One task of this book is to highlight the importance of judgement of this kind within mental health care.

Consider, then, an example discussed at length by Wittgenstein: the 'plus 2' series, the series of numbers produced by starting at 0 and adding 2 sequentially. Having been suitably taught, children are able to carry this series on to arbitrarily high numbers. They can be said to understand the series, to have grasped it. Such understanding is ascribed despite what might seem to be a lack of evidence: the series—and thus the competence—is infinite, whilst the ascription is based on only finite past practice. According to one commentator on Wittgenstein's work, John McDowell, we tend to think of competence in continuing such a series as resulting from a psychological mechanism, which reliably delivers the right result at each point. The misleading thought is this: postulating a psychological mechanism could explain why just the *right* numbers—out of the multitude of potential wrong numbers—are given for an infinite series. This picture can also be augmented, especially in mathematical cases, with the idea that the mechanism tracks or follows objective, perhaps supernatural, rails that are already out there, independently of us. Our continuing a series is merely going over, in bolder pencil, moves already made.

With this assumption in place then it seems that understanding any genuine concept can be codified by giving the principle or formula 'that specifies the conditions under which the concept, in the use of it that one has mastered, is correctly applied' (McDowell 1998b: 62). This is a mistaken view that leads in turn to the assumption that all genuinely cognitive judgements must be governed by an explicit rule:

> Now it is only this misconception of the deductive paradigm that leads us to suppose that the operations of any specific conception of rationality in a particular area—any specific conception of what counts as doing the same thing—must be deductively explicable; that is, that there must be a formulable universal principle suited to serve as major premiss in syllogistic explanations ... (McDowell 1998b: 62)

Thus, it seems that anything that fails to pass this test is not a case of genuine concept application or conceptual judgement. So if value judgement is a candidate for rule governed or conceptualised judgement it should, it seems, be codifiable. If it is not codifiable then it is not rational judgement either.

This line of argument rests on a mistake, however. It goes wrong in the assumption that it is necessary, or even helpful, to postulate a psychological mechanism to explain an ability to follow a rule. Postulating such a state of mind is an 'idle wheel' because it cannot ground the kind of expectation that either we, or other people, will continue in the same (successful) way. As Wittgenstein argues, if a direct inference from how someone has made judgements in the past to their future judgements were not reliable, postulating an intervening mechanism would not help either. In the case of ascribing understanding to others, past practice, once described as mere *inductive* evidence for a mechanism, could be evidence for any number of diverging mechanisms. The same practice could be interpreted as being in accord with any number of different mechanisms (or 'bent' rules in the terminology of Chapter 1).

In the first person case there is a problem in specifying the right mechanism to embody. Any real causal mechanism might misfire or breakdown and, thus, cannot be used to specify the correct continuation of the series. Any abstract representation of a mechanism, or any specification of the series using symbols, will require the correct interpretation which will beg the question.

As will be further discussed in Chapters 4 and 6, a key move to avoid this problem is to reject the idea that an interpretation mediates between understanding subjects and the application of rules they make. In the third person case, the ascription of understanding to others is not based on theory neutral evidence: a description of past practice that is 'agnostic' between different possible rules. Instead, as long as one adopts the same perspective, then one can see in someone else's practice the rule that is exemplified. That we are able to adopt the same perspective depends on the fact that we share many background interests, habits, dispositions, preferences and interests or the same 'whirl of organism' in Stanley Cavell's memorable phrase (Cavell 1969: 52).

In the first person case, the important lesson is that the capacity to self-ascribe understanding is not based on an interpretation of inner mental signs and symbols.

Rather, it is a primitive, but fallible ability, which cannot be decomposed into more basic mental processes or mechanisms.

Thus, even in the case of a judgement that can be codified—by the axioms of Peano arithmetic, for example—the principle itself has to be applied through a kind of practical judgement. Whatever principles can be used to encode such practice, their application relies on practical judgements, which are not themselves codified.

Wittgenstein's discussion should undermine the prejudice that wherever there is a rational judgement, it must be encoded in a principle, since principles themselves cannot govern judgement unaided. Without the prejudice, however, there is no reason to doubt the appearance that value judgements are made without a close framework of principles.

## Overview of the model of values that underpins values-based practice

The view of values-based practice set out above is thus one in which there is a sharp separation of facts and values, as an instance of a broader distinction between the normative and non-normative, the space of reasons and the realm of law. It does not, however, subscribe to a widespread subjectivism about values. I have maintained some agnosticism about the status of values and only argued that one influential argument against their objectivity fails. VBP is, however, committed to the uncodifiability of values: value judgements cannot be given an algorithmic specification.

How radical an approach is values-based practice? It is certainly radical in its theoretical foundations, drawing as it does on the resources not of substantive ethical theories, such as consequentialism and deontology, but on analytic philosophy, specifically the linguistic-analytic Oxford school of the middle decades of the 20th century, and subsequent occasional exemplars, such as Hilary Putnam. It has also (as noted briefly above) been remarkably effective at a practical level, in driving developments in training, research and service delivery in mental health. But how *radical* an approach is it in its applications to practice? The answer to this depends on with what views of the relationship of clinical judgement, medical ethics and the possibility of a value-free medical science core for diagnosis it is compared. On the conventional view, good clinical judgement is based on the combination of a purely scientific, value free, diagnosis coupled with and governed by the requirements of medical ethics, codified in a set of principles. The combination of a purely descriptive view of science underpinning clinical judgements is, for example, found in Beauchamp and Childress' *Principles of Biomedical Ethics*.

In 'Psychiatric ethics: a biological ugly duckling?' Bill Fulford and Tony Hope, an Oxford-based ethicist, examine the application of the Four Principles approach to judgements about compulsory psychiatric treatment. Whilst praising some aspects of the analysis they argue that:

> there are clear indications that a scientific model of the medical concepts is implicit in Beauchamp and Childress' *Principles*. There are hints of this in repeated references to the pre-eminence of the doctor's specialist knowledge: autonomy can mean acceptance of authority; the authority of the doctor is modelled on that of a parent; a patient's (autonomous) wishes may be overridden where these amount to 'poor choices about courses of action recommended by their physicians'. The most explicit indication, however, comes in the discussion of rationality, which like other elements of competence, often involves references to (highly contestable) value judgements about what a rational person would do. But they then go on to contrast the evaluative nature of judgements of rationality with medical judgements. Balancing autonomy with beneficence is said to be a 'moral *not a medical* problem'. Moreover, 'if precise, non-evaluative criteria were available for making such determinations of competence, the [problem of deciding whether someone's choices are rational] would vanish'; as it is 'moral judgements and policy choices ... cannot be avoided'. All this suggests, then, that Beauchamp and Childress assume a standard 'medical' model of the medical concepts in which they are, at root, value-free. (Fulford and Hope 1994: 688–9)

So the implication is that, against the conventional view, values-based practice is radical because it is based on the view that values are present in *diagnosis*, as well as treatment and thus there is no value-free scientific core, at least as defined by disease concepts. Of course, according to the model, there is a clear descriptive aspect of medical science corresponding to the descriptive parts of biological and other sciences. VBP, as Fulford has put it, is a values-added not science-subtracted approach (see also Chapter 1). The extension of values into diagnosis, broadly defined as how a subject's problems are understood, is foundational to values-based practice. In this respect, Fulford's analysis is complementary to the detailed work of the American psychiatrist John Sadler, charting the rich variety of values that are evident throughout the categories in the American Psychiatric Association's classification of mental disorders, the *Diagnostic and Statistical Manual* (Sadler 2004). All the same, it would be possible to adopt all the principles of VBP except, crucially, the first one, if one has reason to adopt a values-out position in the debate about diagnosis, but still thinks that treatment or management answers to values are best handled along these lines.

What of the further aspect of the conventional view that the values that have to be added to a value-free scientific core are encoded in quasi-legal ethical principles? As described in the first section of this chapter, there is a rich literature in bioethics exploring a diverse range of theoretical approaches to ethics. Some of these are explicitly based on principles. Others, such as virtue ethics, narrative ethics and casuistry play down the role of principles. In the final section of this chapter, however, I will examine Beauchamp and Childress' Four Principles approach. The reason for this is two-fold. First, it is very influential in practice, perhaps because it seems to balance specific concrete guidance and flexibility. Secondly, however, the Four Principles approach raises the question of what can and cannot be codified in ethical judgement. Whilst Beauchamp and Childress stress that their Four Principles approach is not simply algorithmic, it can seem that way in practice in a way that VBP, for example, surely could not. Furthermore, this misreading of the Four Principles is encouraged by its failure to give an account of the metaphysics of values. The final section of this chapter will thus examine the presuppositions of the Four Principles approach in order both to highlight the central importance of uncodified judgement in mental health care and also to fill out the view of values it presupposes.

## 3. The role of judgement in the Four Principles approach to medical ethics

Although Beauchamp and Childress' *Principles of Biomedical Ethics* stresses the need for judgement in coming to ethically informed clinical decisions, there is a danger that, in practice, clinicians can come to think of the Four Principles as a kind of algorithmic method. The final section of this chapter will examine the cause of this impression: the absence of a proper account of the *metaphysics* of values. Usefully for medical ethics teaching, *Principles of Biomedical Ethics* stresses the practical use of the Four Principles for *guiding* judgements: the epistemology (the study of knowledge) of values. In this case, however, a little more metaphysics or ontology (the study of what exists) should have a positive effect on practice.

The first subsection sets out the bare bones of the Four Principles approach drawing out those aspects of *Principles of Biomedical Ethics*, which encourage the criticism mentioned above. The aim is not to give a balanced reading so much as a typical reading. Next, I argue that if the emphasis on the guidance of moral judgement is augmented by a 'particularist' account of the metaphysics of values then the danger of an algorithmic interpretation can be reduced. Finally, I consider how much the resultant picture diverges from Beauchamp and Childress' aim.

### A closer look at the Four Principles approach

The Four Principles approach, in Tom Beauchamp and James Childress' *Principles of Biomedical Ethics*, is, to a first approximation, a principles-based approach to ethics or a form of 'principlism'. Ethical judgements are informed by principles in a 'top-down' manner (Beauchamp and Childress 2001: 385). One of the contrasts to this is a bottom-up or case-based approach.

The authors' principlism is indebted to the work of the early 20th century British philosopher W. D. Ross. They say that he had 'more influence on the present authors than any twentieth century writer' (Beauchamp and Childress 2001: 402) and in particular: 'Ross' distinction between *prima facie* and *actual* obligations is basic for our analysis' (Beauchamp and Childress 2001: 14).

According to Ross, moral duties are encoded in general principles. Each principle imposes a '*prima facie*' duty: a duty that would be obligatory all other things being equal, that is if no other principles were to apply. Whilst the principles encode *prima facie* duties, the obligation to act in a particular situation requires an actual or concrete duty: the all-things-considered duty imposed by the situation as a whole. This turns on the interplay of the principles—possibly a subset of them—that are relevant to the case, but because the different principles can pull in different directions the actual duty depends on which duty, in the situation, is the strongest.

Ross himself proposed seven such duties: fidelity, reparation, gratitude, non-maleficence beneficence, self-improvement and justice. Beauchamp and Childress' Four Principles—beneficence, non-maleficence, autonomy and justice—are a smaller number of universal duties more relevant to medicine. Nevertheless, even with this smaller number, the principles can conflict.

Since this is a form of principlism, if the principles conflict then some method of determining the actual duty that they underpin should be available. Beauchamp and Childress describe two methods for coping with conflict between principles: specification and balancing. (Ross himself does not offer an account. This is the basis of a criticism of him by the contemporary moral philosopher Jonathan Dancy (Dancy 1993: 98).)

Specification is way of deriving more concrete guidance from the fairly abstract higher level principles. It is described in outline thus:

> Specification is a process of reducing the indeterminateness of abstract norms and providing them with action guiding content. For example, without further specification, do no harm is an all-too-bare starting point for thinking through problems, such as assisted suicide and euthanasia. It will not adequately guide action when norms conflict. (Beauchamp and Childress 2001: 16)

This looks at first to be a kind of deduction. Much as, once particular assumptions are made, Kepler's Laws of planetary motion can be (more or less) derived from Newtonian physics, so a specified rule can be derived from a higher level principle. Just as Kepler's Laws are useful in the specific context of planetary systems so a specified principle—such as that doctors should put their patients' interests first—can be tailored to give concrete guidance to cases of, for example, euthanasia.

Although specification is some form of derivation, however, it cannot strictly be deduction because 'specified' lower level rules have more content than the principles from which they are drawn. The validity of deductive inference, by contrast, is underpinned by the fact that a conclusion cannot contain information that was not already in the premises. Since specification is amplifiable—more content is generated—it cannot be deductive. Nevertheless, however precisely the four principles give rise to more concrete specifications in rules, the rules arrived at help generate actual duties when applied to concrete situations.

What is more, Beauchamp and Childress suggest that specification can dissolve an apparent conflict between principles by narrowing the scope of the principles in play. Two specific rules derived from principles that, in a particular circumstance, appear to conflict, may themselves be consistent. Specification thus fits the general aim of principlism: to encode moral guidance in general norms (principles and rules in the terminology here). So far, too, it appears to underpin an algorithmic approach to moral judgements. Armed with suitable specifications, actual duties can be derived robotically.

The second tool for generating an actual duty from apparently conflicting principles is, in principle, less algorithmic. It is called 'balancing' and complements specification thus:

> Principles, rules and rights require *balancing* no less than *specification*. We need both methods because each addresses a dimension of moral principles and rules: *range and scope*, in the case of specification, and *weight or strength*, in the case of balancing. Specification entails a substantive refinement of the range and scope of norms, whereas balancing consists of deliberation and judgement about the relative weights or strengths of norms. Balancing is especially important for reaching judgements in individual cases. (Beauchamp and Childress 2001: 18)

In fact, despite the talk of deliberation and judgement here, Beauchamp and Childress go on to specify six conditions that have to apply before one principle can be taken to outweigh another ('1. Better reasons can be offered to act on the overriding norm than on the infringed norm ... 2. The moral objective justifying the infringement must have a realistic prospect of achievement', etc. (Beauchamp and Childress 2001: 19–20)). In other words, they deploy a further codification which plays down the role of individual judgement or sensitivity to the case. The suggestion is that the list of conditions is needed to protect ethics from 'purely intuitive or subjective judgement' (Beauchamp and Childress 2001: 21).

Nevertheless, Beauchamp and Childress do still suggest that balancing requires a degree of judgement (in the non-algorithmic sense I intend), which goes beyond the codifications they provide. They also think that there will be genuine moral dilemmas that remain after the principles have been deployed calling, instead, for an exercise of judgement, but it is all too easy to lose sight of the role of judgement in both medical ethical teaching and in discussions of the Four Principles approach in journals.

One problem is this: standard cases come to dominate teaching and discussion. Thus, for example, the case of the Jehovah's Witness who competently refuses life threatening treatment is taken to exemplify the conflict of beneficence and autonomy and, on the standard solution, autonomy is taken rightly to dominate (cf. Beauchamp 2003; Macklin 2003). (Things differ in the standard case of his or her young child.) The case is sketched in abstract and ideal terms, and becomes, itself, a kind of rule to be applied to further actual cases. Competence in solving standard cases, in applying the principles and giving them standardly approved weight, becomes second nature to medical students keen to pass their ethics course and the element of individual judgement is downplayed.

A second problem is this: there is no clear account of what kind of skill is involved in balancing principles. Beauchamp and Childress express the worry that, if balancing is not itself subject to further guidelines, it will be merely subjective. This seems to suggest that if balancing is not an expression of mere subjective whimsy it must somehow be guided by principles in an inchoate way, which again suggests that it is really an algorithmic matter.

In summary, a cursory reading of *Principles of Biomedical Ethics* together with the needs of medical ethics teaching encourages an algorithmic approach and hides the element of skilled uncodified judgement involved. Beauchamp and Childress concentrate on a top-down approach that seems to dictate almost deductively ('almost' because specification is amplifiable) actual duties. Their worry is that when principles cannot be given there is a danger of subjectivism. All this encourages the worry with which I began, but it can naturally be eased by thinking a little more about what is being decided when conflicting principles are balanced.

## Adding an account of the metaphysics of values

In this subsection I will suggest that a particularist view of the metaphysics of values helps ease the worry that the Four Principles approach is algorithmic in practice and examine how close this actually fits the *Principles of Biomedical Ethics* in the final subsection.

Beauchamp and Childress introduce the Four Principles primarily as a tool to offer guidance for medical ethics. They say 'These principles can … function as guidelines for professional ethics' (Beauchamp and Childress 2001: 12). The emphasis of the book is practical—on specifying duties in the light of the principles—but in moral philosophy in general guidance is only one role for principles in a broadly principlist approach to moral values. (Ross himself, in fact, does not suggest that principles do play a guiding role.)

In addition to asking what *guides* moral judgement one should also ask what *disciplines* it? What, in other words, makes the difference between a judgement being correct or incorrect? This is not to ask how we know whether a judgement is correct, but rather what, possibly underlying, standard makes the difference. Whilst the question of guidance is an epistemological question, the question of discipline is ontological and helps characterise what sort of judgements are in play.

Putting aside the subtleties of recent moral philosophy, there are three broad answers to this second question.

### Nothing

If nothing disciplines ethical judgements, then there is no difference between right and wrong, correct and incorrect. Beauty, on a popular view, is like this. If beauty is merely in the eye of the beholder, then what is in the eye answers to nothing and there is nothing that disciplines that response. Beauty is nothing substantial.

There may be philosophical reasons to adopt this view. Some philosophers are driven to it because they find neither of the other answers set out below plausible. Some neo-Humean philosophers take the surface form of ethical judgement to be systematically erroneous, others that it, at least, requires reinterpretation. In the context of medical ethics, however, there is also a practical justification for rejecting this approach. If one of the aims of medical ethics teaching is to foster respect for genuine constraints on clinical judgement, it will hardly help to promote an error theory of ethics.

### Principles

What makes the movement of a chess piece, its bare displacement along a vector, a chess move, a legitimate action within the game? A necessary (but not sufficient) element of the answer is its accord with the rules of chess. Those rules or norms set the standard of correctness for moves and, thus, partly constitute a move. Chess is merely a human institution, but a similar approach is plausible in the case of arithmetic judgements whether the rules are taken to be the informal rules in which elementary students are drilled (such as the rules about carrying over the tens) or the logical formalisation in Peano's axioms.

In both these cases, rules or principles function as *epistemological* guides. To determine whether to believe that a movement is a legitimate chess move or what the answer to an arithmetic sum is one can look to the rules. However, the rules also determine what correctness comprises and thus the *ontology* of chess and maths, chess or maths 'facts'. (The former includes such facts as that rooks cannot move diagonally; the latter that seven plus five equals twelve.) Because they answer to consistent rules, these facts can be marshalled into deductive structures.

According to principlism in ethics, ethical principles serve both these functions. As well as guiding moral judgements, they set the standard of correctness and incorrectness for those judgements, but this raises a substantial challenge. If principles discipline judgements, then they should be able to meet two constraints:

- ◆ they should give the right sort of guidance to resemble *moral* principles, and
- ◆ they should be consistent.

The problem is that these two constraints pull in opposite directions.

If there is only one principle then meeting the second constraint is not difficult. A single universal principle, such as Kant's categorical imperative, can be self-consistent, but it does not seem to capture the whole of moral reasoning. In a practical situation it is simply not clear what substantive advice can be derived from 'Act only according to that maxim by which you can at the same time will that it should become a universal law', whilst the derivation of more specific guidelines for every situation looks none too easy.

Beauchamp and Childress, following Ross, argue that the only realistic approach to meet the first constraint is to accept that there are a number of principles that govern moral judgement. But, as they realise, the principles conflict. If they are to serve the role of disciplining moral judgements, such conflict is more than just an epistemological complexity. It threatens the idea that all that makes a moral judgement correct or incorrect is accord with a set of principles. Something else is needed to explain how to balance the principles in the face of a particular situation: what the *aim* of balancing is.

## Particulars themselves

If not 'nothing' and not 'accord with principles' what answer can we give to the question: what disciplines a judgement? A third candidate is 'the facts'. Given the general contrast of fact and value discussed so far, that answer may not seem promising here. Nevertheless, the idea is that, rather than thinking that a particular situation merely prompts a balancing of conflicting principles which themselves discipline a judgement, one should think that the aim of the judgement is just to get the situation itself right.

On this third view, the situation itself contains evaluative features—values— and ethical judgement aims to describe these. This view is called 'particularism'. There are a number of philosophical objections to a particularist view of ethical judgement. One is that it requires accepting that the world itself is partly made up of features that can only be understood from a particular standpoint. This runs counter to the idea that what is really real, what is 'out there', requires no special perspective to understand it. As the philosopher Thomas Nagel points out (albeit critically), one feature of the progress of science has been a move away from descriptions of the world which depend on a having particular perspective, or particular sensory apparatus, to a description as from nowhere (Nagel 1986). According to moral particularism, the world contains evaluatively charged features the comprehension and detection of which requires the development of a kind of moral sensibility.

A second philosophical objection turns on the particularist claim that beliefs about evaluative features of a situation can motivate action by themselves, without any additional desire. This runs counter to a long standing assumption that action is explained by a practical syllogism, which contains both beliefs *and desires*.

Nevertheless, whilst both of these present *prima facie* difficulties they can at least be addressed. The first objection can be addressed by diagnosing the influence of the methods of science not only for explaining and predicting events governed by natural laws, but also as a metaphysical touchstone for what is really real. The second objection can be addressed in a similar way. It is a similar piece of scientism to assume that the world cannot contain motivational factors (see, for example, McDowell 1998b: 50–73, 131–150, discussed in Thornton 2004: 63–99).

The advantage of particularism is that it helps provide a context for balancing principles in the Four Principles approach. These can now be seen merely as guides to judgement which itself aims to get the evaluative features of concrete situations right. The situations, rather than a combination of principles, make the judgements right or wrong. As mere guides, principles can be more or less useful depending on the situation at hand, but as reminders of the kind of factors that it is useful to take note of—think of the autonomy of the subjects involved, avoid harm and so on—they have a role both in practice and education. (The idea that principles serve as reminders is developed in Dancy 1993: 67.)

It may seem that particularism is a method without content for medical ethics. What specific guidance can it offer? It is worth comparing with two other aspects of clinical judgement both of which concern the gathering of data, the signs and symptoms presented by a patient. In that context, there are some guidelines and even a partial codification of diagnosis in the hypothetico-deductive model (Elstein *et al.* 1978). Nevertheless, even in the case of physical medicine, the guidelines are not taken to constitute the phenomena in question. They are epistemic tools designed to help get clinical judgements about particular patients right. In mental health care, diagnosis is also taken to include gaining an understanding of patients' beliefs and experiences. There is little by way of guidelines for how to rationalise life experiences yet, nevertheless, this is taken to be a legitimate clinical skill. Moral particularism takes the reasons for moral judgements to be equally uncodifiable, although principles can help serve as reminders for what might be relevant, whilst at the same time concerning real features of situations.

Why would this emphasis on the values realised in particular situations help avoid the risk that the application of the Four Principles is, in practice, algorithmic? Because it reduces the idea that moral judgement is a closed 'game' with a limited number of factors to be addressed. Making real situations central to the actual practice of ethical skill and principles secondary encourages a realistic view of the complexity of judgement. Situations are not merely constituted by the interplay of the Four Principles, but rather predate and test those principles.

It also encourages a critical approach to the Four Principles themselves. Perhaps there are better tools to chart the space of values than just those principles. Whilst Beauchamp and Childress are open to this possibility to the extent that they see the need to defend their view, it risks being lost in medical ethics teaching and subsequent practice.

In this section I have suggested that the Four Principles approach is usually explicitly introduced as an answer to the question of what guides or should guide ethical judgement, but that in the wider area of moral philosophy, principlism is also supposed to answer the more fundamental question of what disciplines such judgement. Principlism has difficulty answering this question because of the dual challenge of showing that the principles selected capture sufficiently what we pre-philosophically mean by ethical judgement but also that they are consistent. By giving a different answer to the 'discipline question' we can sidestep this problem and, at the same time, reduce the temptation to construe the Four Principles approach as circumventing the need for judgement.

## Is particularism consistent with the Four Principles approach?

In the previous section I distinguished between two questions to which moral particularism might be an answer. One was 'what guides ethical claims?', the other 'what disciplines them?'. I outlined the attractions of a particularist answer to the second and suggested that it also helps emphasise the central role of good judgement in medical ethics. In this section, I will return to the question of guidance in order to clarify the nature of particularism, and to explore its relation to what Beauchamp and Childress themselves say about 'bottom-up' approaches.

According to the philosopher Ben Smith, in a recent *Journal of Medical Ethics* paper:

> Moral particularism can be understood as propounding a 'case-by-case' methodology in dealing with moral questions ...
>
> What motivates particularism ... is hostility to the manner in which agents tend to deliberate about a particular case as though it must be considered always and only with reference to a relevant principle ... The moral particularist complains that this 'intellectual' way of reaching a moral conclusion can serve to obscure the potential complexity of the particular case. (Smith 2002: 244)

This summary emphasises guidance rather than discipline. Ethical judgements, according to particularism, should be guided by close attention to the case at hand, rather than by appeal to principles. According to the most influential recent exponent of particularism, the UK philosopher Jonathan Dancy:

> The primary focus of particularism is the particular case, not surprisingly. This means that one's main duty, in moral judgement, is to look really closely at the case before one. Our first question is not 'Which other cases does this one best resemble?', but rather 'What is the nature of the case before us?'. (Dancy 1993: 63)

In other words, in addition to the idea that judgements are made right or wrong by reference to the situation, rather than reference to principles, principles also have (and should have) little role in deliberation. How different is this approach from the combination I suggested in the previous section: a principles-based account of guidance and a situation-based account of discipline?

Dancy argues for a radical difference. He argues, against the moral philosophy of W. D. Ross on which Beauchamp and Childress' Four Principles approach is based, that principles do not succeed even in capturing *prima facie* duties. In appropriate circumstances, a principle that apparently encodes a *prima facie* duty can invert its normal force or 'valency'. Consider the idea that, all other things being equal, promoting happiness is an ethical good. Now imagine two equally competent dentists who both scrupulously minimise patient discomfort and cause only the same small unavoidable amount. One of them, however, takes great pleasure in her patients' pain. To whom should a practice manager favour sending patients? According to some ethical intuitions, one should not promote the psychotic dentist's happiness. If so promoting happiness has the opposite valence to normal. The dentist's pleasure is a reason against sending patients to him or her. Dancy claims that, therefore, Ross' idea that actual duties are forged from *prima facie* duties, which always have the same 'all other things being equal' force, is mistaken.

Dancy's emphasis on the particular case, however, threatens to become too radical. Without at least conceptual connections between one case and another, individual cases look like an instance of what Wilfrid Sellars terms the Myth of the Given (Sellars 1997). It looks as though experience of a particular case might be supposed to comprise a foundation for judgement that is independent of all other judgements, but Sellars has convincingly argued that the Myth of the Given is untenable. So the question is: is there a middle ground between the rejection of moral principles encoding *prima facie* duties and the rejection of moral concepts that enable one to judge that one case is relevantly similar to another? I will not attempt to adjudicate that debate here. (For a general assessment, see Hooker and Little 2000; see also Smith 2003; for a defence of the use of analogy in ethical judgement against Dancy's particularism, see Smith 2002.) However, examination of the motivation for Dancy's particularism suggests that there need not be a problem.

Dancy's main argument for particularism is what he calls 'holism in the theory of reasons'. He argues that:

> The leading thought behind particularism is the thought that the behaviour of a reason (or of a consideration that serves as a reason) in a new case cannot be predicted from its behaviour elsewhere. The way in which the consideration functions *here* either will or at least may be affected by other considerations here present. So there is no ground for the hope that we can find out here how that consideration functions *in general*, somehow, nor for the hope that we can move in any smooth way to how it will function in a different case. (Dancy 1993: 60)

Although this is not Dancy's argument, an analogy with a different area of philosophy helps illustrate the main point.

In recent philosophy of mind, two opposing views have dominated the problem of other minds: how we can know one another's mental states. These are called 'theory theory' and 'simulation theory'. According to the former, we have knowledge of other minds through a theory of mind. In much the way that a theory mediates between observation of patterns in a cloud chamber and a judgement of the underlying particles causing them, so a theory of mind mediates between observed behaviour and underlying mental states (Fodor and Chihara 1965). According to simulation theory, by contrast, things are not so intellectual. One need merely imaginatively put oneself into another person's predicament and see what mental states one would form oneself (Heal 1995). On this view, one need merely possess a mind, not a theory of mind, to know another's mind. The debate is not as clear cut as this, however, because, to be plausible, the theory proposed by theory theorists need merely be tacitly known and, if so, perhaps the ability to simulate is describable in such a theory. Thus, the two sides may be closer than they at first appeared.

Nevertheless, there remains one reason to hold that the approaches are distinct and thus that the ability to simulate cannot be encoded in a theory. Imagining oneself in another's situation requires, in addition to thinking of their motives and desires, assessing what it would be rational to believe in that case in the light of their other beliefs. This requires assessing the interplay of reasons in context. Whilst there may be guidelines that help govern beliefs in some areas they will in general be sensitive to other factors. A cow-like visual appearance may usually indicate the presence of a cow. That might approach the status of a principle. However, in the context of antecedent reason—perhaps a well-founded general zoological theory—to believe that there are no cows present, but there are other similar animals or replicas, that principle will no longer hold.

Simulation theory is thus a form of particularism. It denies that reasons can, in general, be governed by principles, but it need not require an epistemological foundation—an experiential intake that does not also depend on one's other beliefs. Imaginatively putting oneself into someone else's position—both literally and figuratively—requires imagining how the world looks from there. That involves an exercise of judgement concerning the interplay of reasons available, but it does not imply any form of 'Given'. By analogy there seems no reason to think that particularist judgement in the ethical case need subscribe to that myth either.

How does such a moderate epistemological particularism fit with what Beauchamp and Childress themselves say about bottom-up approaches? They focus on Albert Jonsen and Stephen Toulmin's casuistry, which they characterise as a focus on an 'intimate acquaintance with particular situations and the historical record of similar cases' (Beauchamp and Childress 2001: 393). This fits the sketch of particularism given above, but unlike radical particularism at least, casuistry relies heavily on reasoning by analogy. 'The leading cases—often called paradigm cases—become the most enduring and authoritative sources of appeal in the underlying consensus ... Decisions reached about moral rights and wrongs in these seminal cases serve as a form of authority for new cases' (Beauchamp and Childress 2001: 394). They go on to criticise it, saying that it is a 'method without content' (Beauchamp and Childress 2001: 395) and that it requires ethical principles to serve as the initial premises for analogical reasoning. As a result, they suggest a combined approach: 'Principles need to be made specific for cases, and case analysis needs illumination from general principles' (Beauchamp and Childress 2001: 397). (This is why their position is principlist only to a first approximation.)

What do they mean by this? Normally, combining opposing philosophical positions risks contradiction, but given the distinction between the questions of guidance and discipline sketched above, it is possible to suggest in more detail than Beauchamp and Childress themselves provide what this might involve. A particularist answer to the discipline question can be combined with a principlist answer to the guidance question. Since the questions are independent, the result is consistent.

In fact, however, the position need not be made up in quite that neat way. A particularist answer to the latter—discipline—question can be combined with a position that is neither strongly particularist nor principlist with regard to the former question of guidance. The analogy with the problem of other minds helps fill this out, whilst reinforcing the need for good judgement. Being responsive to ethically complex situations requires being sensitive to the demands of moral reasons. This involves, in part, working out the combined effect of different factors that are in play at the same time. Principles may help in this. They can serve as reminders of factors that can be important (Dancy 1993: 67). However, just as we do not form reasons for belief in accord with an explicit or implicit theory of best evidential practice, so good ethical judgement turns on a skilled intellectual appreciation of the case at hand. The price of emphasising the central importance of good judgement in medical ethics is distinguishing between the question of guidance and discipline and adopting a particularist ontology in response to the latter.

## 4. Conclusions

Medical ethics is both practically and conceptually complex. Even in the comparatively stable area of high level moral theory or normative ethics, there remain a number of competing theories, relying on competing intuitions, about how judgements should be guided by ethical values. Even if a justified choice can be made of the best such high level ethical theory, complexities remain about how it is to be applied in practice. The details of a particular clinical situation have to be correctly captured in appropriate language and then the correct judgement derived. In principles-based approaches, this involves either balancing opposing principles or deriving from a single principle relevant concrete guidance. In a consequentialist framework, the nature of the consequences have to be estimated. In virtue ethics, the choices of a virtuous agent have to be determined.

In addition to those general conceptual problems, psychiatry adds further difficulties. On the one hand, mental health care sometimes involves compulsory detention and treatment of fully conscious adults. This practice calls for philosophical analysis and justification and it goes to the heart of the nature of mental illness.

On the other, mental health care presents a broader range of conflicting values than other areas of medicine which have, somehow, to be managed. In the UK, a skills-based approach for dealing with conflicting values in medicine has recently been developed to help guide clinical judgements under the name 'values-based practice'. I have argued in this chapter that a key to values-based practice is the uncodifiablity of values. It is this that requires the need for judgement in the sense it has in the phrase 'having good judgement'. That, indeed, is why approaches to mental health care that follow the principles of VBP focus on the development of clinical skills.

In the final section, I have examined the Four Principles approach to medical ethical judgements. Notwithstanding the range of rival approaches, the Four Principles approach is very influential in medical practice, perhaps because it combines rules to guide ethical judgement with a degree of flexibility. Nevertheless, whilst its authors stress that it is not intended to be algorithmic, it can be interpreted in that way. Closer attention, however, to the constraints on any principles-based approach to ethics suggests that, contrary to first appearances, the Four Principles approach shares with VBP a key need for good judgement in assessing a particular situation. Whilst principles can serve as useful reminders of what should be taken into account in framing an ethical judgement, the approach is best understood as a form of moral particularism, suggesting a need for judgement in charting the real values that help make up the social world.

Part II

# Meanings

Chapter 3

# Understanding psychopathology

## Plan of the chapter

Psychiatry, unlike other branches of medicine, concerns meanings as much as physiological facts. Central to psychiatry is the aim of *understanding* individuals, as much as *explaining* their illnesses, but understanding meaning is, on the face of it, a different kind of intelligibility from framing causal, aetiological explanations. This chapter and the next will explore the role of understanding meaning in psychiatry.

The first part of the chapter outlines Jaspers' views on the centrality of understanding for psychopathology and thus for psychiatry. I will begin with a biographical sketch (based on work by the UK psychiatrist Chris Walker (Fulford *et al.* 2006: 166–7)) and then look more closely at two papers published in 1912 and 1913: 'The phenomenological approach in psychopathology' (Jaspers (1912) 1968) and 'Causal and "meaningful" connections between life history and psychosis' (Jaspers (1913) 1974). These two papers are clear statements of Jaspers' views of what he calls static understanding or phenomenology, and genetic understanding. These are both forms of empathy that Jaspers compares with transferring oneself into someone else's psyche. The first concerns the intrinsic nature of mental states and experiences. The second concerns the way one state gives rise to another, ideally and typically. I will end the first section by explaining Jaspers' view that, although understanding lies at the heart of psychiatry, there are, nevertheless, limits on its range. Some phenomena remain incomprehensible.

The second half of the chapter looks at recent philosophical models of delusion which aim to expand the horizons of understanding and thus to provide a kind of empathic insight into psychopathological symptoms. I will examine accounts based on Brendan Maher, Louis Sass, John Campbell, Martin Davies and Richard Gipps.

This is a developing area of the philosophy of psychiatry and the examples given are intended to illustrate the wide variety of approaches possible. Nevertheless, they also illustrate the very real difficulty in providing a general route to understanding delusion. The best that may be hoped is that a plurality of perspectives can help a case by case partial insight into the experiences of sufferers. There may be no short cut to good clinical judgement.

## 1. Jaspers on the role of understanding in psychiatry

### Biographical sketch of Jaspers

Karl Jaspers was born in 1883. He studied first law and then medicine at university, graduating as a doctor in 1908 when he started to work as an assistant in the department of psychiatry in the University of Heidelberg. Kraepelin's influential textbook of psychiatry was in its eighth edition at this time. As a young man he read widely, studying not only medicine, but psychology and philosophy, and it was the depth of his philosophical understanding which equipped him to make his unique contributions to psychiatry.

Jaspers' professor in the Heidelberg Department of Psychiatry was Franz Nissl: a neurohistologist who discovered the dye that allowed the structure of nerve cells to be clearly seen for the first time. Using this technique, he showed that the neurohistological changes in general paralysis were different to the changes described by Alois Alzheimer in dementia. General paralysis was a degenerative dementia, which had swept Europe after the wars of the late nineteenth century. It was shortly to prove to be a form of neurosyphylis. These were dramatic discoveries, therefore, and the young Jaspers was impressed with Nissl as a scientist. When it came to *clinical* work, however, Jaspers was considerably less impressed.

Psychiatry at the turn of the century in Germany had moved out of the large institutions into university clinics. There was considerable resentment among the institutional psychiatrists that their discipline had been taken over by academic neuroscientists whose knowledge of clinical psychiatry was scant and whom they perceived as being under the spell of a crudely natural scientific model, epitomised by the German psychiatrist Wilhelm Griesinger's famous aphorism 'Mental illnesses are brain illnesses' (Jaspers 1997: 459). Psychiatric researchers at the time, like Griesinger, Alzheimer, Nissl, Carl Meynert and Theodor Wernicke, were actively searching for the neuropathological changes by which they believed the major psychoses could be characterised. Given their success with general paralysis, hopes were high. Jaspers shared these hopes, but he believed the underlying biological approach had been pushed too far. 'These anatomical constructions, however, became quite fantastic (e.g. Meynert, Wernicke) and have rightly been called "Brain Mythologies"' (Jaspers 1997: 18).

Jaspers' reservations about what he perceived as the excessively natural-scientific approach to psychiatry were driven by his understanding of the philosophical debates about psychology in the late nineteenth century, the so-called *Methodenstreit*. This concerned whether the human sciences (the *Geisteswissenschaften*) should try to emulate their far more successful cousins the natural sciences (*Naturwissenschaften*), or whether they should go their own methodological way. 'Positivists', including John Stuart Mill in England, and both Auguste Comte and Emile Durkheim in France, argued that the human sciences were no different from the natural sciences. Others argued that the human or cultural sciences were different from the natural sciences either in terms of the nature of their subject matter or their methodology or both. The latter, in Germany, included Heinrich Rickert, Wilhelm Dilthey and Wilhelm Windelband, who coined the distinction between idiographic and nomothetic:

> So we may say that the empirical sciences seek in the knowledge of reality either the general in the form of the natural law or the particular in the historically determined form [Gestalt]. They consider in one part the ever enduring form, in the other part the unique content, determined within itself, of an actual happening. The one comprises sciences of law, the other sciences of events; the former teaches what always is, the latter what once was. If one may resort to neologisms, it can be said that scientific thought is in the one case nomothetic, in the other idiographic. If we hold to the customary expressions, we may speak further in this sense of the opposition of the natural science and historical disciplines, provided that we bear in mind that in this methodological sense psychology is by all means to be numbered among the natural sciences. (Windelband (1894) 1998: 13)

Crucially for Jaspers, the German philosopher and sociologist Max Weber was among the latter camp.

Jaspers met Max Weber in 1909. He was invited to join Weber's elite intellectual circle and he quickly became one of Weber's key intellectual antagonists.

Jaspers thought of Weber as the 'Galileo of the human sciences' (Ehrlich *et al.* 1986: 478). Although Weber believed that the human sciences involved a distinctive approach, he believed that sociology, his own discipline, was a hybrid subject, living partly within the natural and partly within the human sciences.

Jaspers regarded psychopathology as Weber regarded sociology. It lay both within the natural sciences, pursuing abnormalities of brain functioning, but also within the human sciences, pursuing the experiences, aims, intentions and subjective meanings of its patients. Of course, at a time when psychiatry was dominated by the 'brain mythologists', Jaspers' major aim was to bring psychiatry back within the ambit of the human sciences. He wanted to balance things up. In Weber's work, therefore, which in turn had drawn on the work of Dilthey, Windelband and Rickert, he saw things falling into place, and much of Weber's social theory—interpretation/understanding, *Evidenz*, ideal types, and so forth—was to find its way into his psychopathology. Sometime later he wrote:

> My article of 1912 and this present book (1913) were greeted as something radically new, although all I had done was to link psychiatric reality with the traditional humanities. Looking back now, it seems astonishing that these had been so forgotten and grown so alien to psychiatry. In this way within the confines of psychopathology there grew a methodological comprehension of something which had always been present, but which was fading out of existence and which appeared in striking reverse, 'through the looking-glass' as it were, in Freud's psychoanalysis—a misunderstanding of itself. The way was clear for scientific consciousness to lay hold on human reality and on man's mental estate, his psychoses included, but there was an immediate need to differentiate the *various modes of understanding*, clarify them and embody them in all *the factual content* available to us. (Jaspers 1997: 302)

The period 1909–1913 was a time of high output for Jaspers. He wrote papers on homesickness, hallucinations, pathological jealousy, phenomenology, and the need for both 'causal' (natural scientific) and 'understandable' (human scientific) connections in psychic life. I will discuss two papers published in this period below: 'The phenomenological approach in psychopathology' and 'Causal and "meaningful" connections between life history and psychosis'. However, the culmination of this burst of output was that, in 1911, he was commissioned by the publisher, Springer, to write a textbook of psychopathology. It was thus that his *General Psychopathology* (*Allgemeine Psychopathologie*) appeared in its 1st edition in 1913.

## Jaspers on phenomenological understanding

In 'The phenomenological approach in psychopathology' (Jaspers (1912) 1968), Jaspers sets out his account of the role within psychopathology for a phenomenological approach. As I will explain shortly, phenomenology is, in

Jaspers' view, a form of static understanding by contrast with what he calls genetic understanding, the subject of the next sub-section, but both forms of understanding have in common that they are attempts to explore subjective, as opposed to objective, symptoms. What is the distinction between subjective and objective? Jaspers describes objective symptoms as follows:

> Objective symptoms include all concrete events that can be perceived by the sense, e.g. reflexes, registrable movements, an individual's physiognomy, his motor activity, verbal expression, written productions, actions and general conduct, etc.; all measurable performances ... It is also usual to include under objective symptoms such features as delusional ideas, falsifications of memory, etc., in other words, the rational contents of what the patient tells us. These, it is true, are not perceived by the senses, but only understood; nevertheless, this 'understanding' is achieved through rational thought, without the help of any empathy into the patient's psyche. (Jaspers (1912) 1968: 1313)

The distinction between what is available to rational thought and to empathy is important, and one to which I will return. It helps form a broader conception of what is objective than would generally be accepted today, but this, in turn, gives rise to a correspondingly narrower sense of 'subjective':

> Objective symptoms can all be directly and convincingly demonstrated to anyone capable of sense-perception and logical thought; but subjective symptoms, if they are to be understood, must be referred to some process which, in contrast to sense percep-tion and logical thought, is usually described by the same term 'subjective'. Subjective symptoms cannot be perceived by the sense-organs, but have to be grasped by trans-ferring oneself, so to say, into the other individual's psyche; that is, by empathy. They can only become an inner reality for the observer by his participating in the other person's experiences, not by any intellectual effort. (Jaspers (1912) 1968: 1313)

Jaspers complains that a purely objective psychology leads 'quite systemati-cally to the elimination of everything that can be called mental or psychic' (Jaspers (1912) 1968: 1313). In order to illustrate what he means, Jaspers refers to the assessment of a patient's fatigue through measurable performances, where 'It is not the feeling of fatigue but "objective fatigue" which is being investigated' (Jaspers (1912) 1968: 1314). This suggests a contrast between objective and measurable aspects of physiology and the subjective aspect of what it is like to be or to feel fatigued. Assessing such subjective symptoms requires a kind of imaginative transference or empathy, which lies at the heart of psychopathology.

Having drawn this distinction between subjective and objective, Jaspers then goes on to characterise the aims of phenomenological psychopathology in the following terms:

> What then are the precise aims of this much-abused subjective psychology? ... It asks itself—speaking quite generally—what does mental experience depend on, what are its consequences, and what relationships can be discerned in it? The answers to these

questions are its special aims ... So before real inquiry can begin it is necessary to identify the specific psychic phenomena which are to be its subject, and form a clear picture of the resemblances and differences between them and other phenomena with which they must not be confused. This preliminary work of representing, defining, and classifying psychic phenomena, pursued as an independent activity, constitutes phenomenology. (Jaspers (1912) 1968: 1314)

Thus, the key aim of phenomenology or static understanding is to identify the specific psychic phenomena that are to be its subject, and form a clear picture of the resemblances and differences between them and other phenomena. How does it set about this task?

We should picture only what is really present in the patient's consciousness; anything that has not really presented itself to his consciousness is outside our consideration. We must set aside all outmoded theories, psychological constructs or materialist mythologies of cerebral processes; we must turn our attention only to that which we can understand as having real existence, and which we can differentiate and describe. This, as experience has shown, is in itself a very difficult task. This particular freedom from preconception which phenomenology demands is not something one possesses from the beginning, but something that is laboriously acquired after prolonged and critical work and much effort—often fruitless—in framing constructs and mythologies. (Jaspers (1912) 1968: 1316)

A key aspect of the task of getting a very clear picture of psychological phenomena is thus to attempt to strip away theoretical descriptions or constructs and to get back to the things themselves, to use a slogan of the philosophical phenomenologist Edmund Husserl (1859–1938; the precise nature of whose influence on Jaspers is contested). Of course, from a modern perspective the aim of a theory-free approach has echoes of the aetiological theory-free approach of DSM-III and its successors. Quite how successful a genuinely theory-free approach can be in the face of arguments as to the essential theory-ladenness of data is a matter of debate (see Fulford *et al.* 2006: 288–315).

So far, Jaspers' discussion has presented the difficulties of the phenomenological method, rather than offering specific guidance as to how it is to be achieved. The most concrete account offered of that in this essay runs as follows:

How then do we proceed when we isolate, characterise and give conceptual form to these psychic phenomena? We cannot portray them, or bring them before our eyes in any way that can be perceived by the senses. We can only guide ourselves by a multiple approach. We have to be led, starting *from the outside*, to a real appreciation of a particular psychic phenomenon by looking at its genesis, the conditions for its appearance, its configurations, its context and possible concrete contents; also by making use of intuitive comparison and symbolization, by directing our observations in whatever ways may suggest themselves (as artists do so penetratingly) ...

[T]he phenomenologist can indicate features and characteristics, and show how they can be distinguished and confusion avoided, all with a view to describing the qualitatively separate psychic data. But he must make sure that those to whom he addresses himself do not simply *think* along with him, but that they *see* along with him. (Jaspers (1912) 1968: 1316)

## Jaspers on genetic understanding

I remarked above that Jaspers distinguishes between two legitimate forms of understanding (of subjective phenomena): static understanding, which he also calls phenomenology, and genetic understanding. In 'The phenomenological approach in psychopathology' he characterises the differences thus:

> 'Genetic understanding' [is] the understanding of the meaningful connections between one psychic experience and another, the 'emergence of the psychic from the psychic'. Now phenomenology itself has nothing to do with this 'genetic understanding' and must be treated as something entirely separate. (Jaspers (1912) 1968: 1322)

What then *is* genetic understanding? A fuller discussion is given in another essay from this period 'Causal and "meaningful" connections between life history and psychosis' (Jaspers (1913) 1974). Again, an important clue comes from the distinction mentioned above between rational connections and those that require empathy. Taking the case of understanding a speaker and understanding what the speaker has said, Jaspers comments:

> The first important differentiation was made by Simnel, who showed the difference between the understanding of *what has been said* from understanding the *speaker*. When the contents of thoughts emerge one from another in accordance with the rules of logic, we understand the connections *rationally*. But if we understand the content of the thoughts as they have arisen out of the moods, wishes, and fears of the person who thought them, we understand the connections psychologically or empathetically. Only the latter can be called 'psychological understanding'. Rational understanding always only enables us to say that a certain rational complex, something which can be understood without any psychology whatever, was the content of a mind; empathic understanding, on the other hand, leads us into the psychic connections themselves. Whereas the rational understanding is only an *aid* to psychology, empathic understanding *is* psychology itself. (Jaspers (1913) 1974: 83)

This fits the earlier quotation in which the rational content of what a patient reports was characterised as an objective symptom. Equally, the rational interconnection between reports, their implications and so forth, is also outside the domain of subjective psychology, but if empathy, in the service of genetic understanding, does not chart the logical or rational connection between one thought and another, what is the basis of such psychological understanding? Jaspers' answer is not entirely clear. He says:

> We experience immediate evidence which we cannot reduce further nor base on any kind of other evidence. (Jaspers (1913) 1974: 84)

> Meaningful connections are ideally typical connections. They are self-evident. (Jaspers (1913) 1974: 85)

In other words, when there is a self-evident connection between one state and another, a connection that is typical, although perhaps not always realised in practice, genetic understanding of it, through empathy, is possible. Realising that one has won the national lottery, and thus solved all one's financial problems might lead, ideally and typically, to a state of happiness. Normally, to explain someone's sudden happiness one might simply and sufficiently say that they have just heard that they have won the national lottery. Of course, in some unusual cases, that might not be a reason for happiness. The normal connection is basic—no more needs to be said—but it need not hold in all cases. It is ideally typical.

Thus, the relationship between static and genetic understanding is like this. The former articulates and vividly presents what it is like, for example, to have a sudden realisation or what it is like to be in a state of happiness. It makes these kinds of state clear for further inquiry prior to the imposition of psychological theory. Genetic understanding adds to this the connection of how one state arises—ideally and typically—from the other. Such connections are shared empathically by psychological subjects including psychiatrists and their patients.

Jaspers' characterisation of static understanding has echoes in a recent debate within the philosophy of mind between 'theory theory' and 'simulation theory' accounts of knowledge of other people's minds (Carruthers and Smith 1996). According to theory theory approaches, access to and thus knowledge of other people's minds is mediated by possession of a theory of mind. The theory is a body of deductively structured generalisations about the unseen causes of observable (speech and other) behaviour. This approach to the epistemological problem of how we can know about other minds thus dovetails with what are called 'functionalist' approaches to the ontological problem of what sort of things mental states are. Functionalism characterises mental states in causal and functional terms mediating between perceptual inputs and behavioural outputs. In other words, according to functionalism mental states are akin to software states running on the brain as a computer. By characterising types of mental state in second order terms, functionalism aims to answer the problem of relating minds and bodies without simply reducing mental states to brain states. Theory theory approaches deploy broadly functionalist characterisations of what mental states are to explain, in addition, how we can have knowledge of them (in the case of other people).

Simulation theory, by contrast, explains knowledge of other minds not by possession of a theory of minds, but merely by possession of a mind itself. The idea is that it is possible to have knowledge of another person's mental states by imaginatively putting oneself into his or her predicament. One 'runs' one's deliberative processes 'off line', as it were. Simulation theory is thus a form of empathy, but, unlike Jaspers' account, there is no restriction to non-rational patterns of thoughts emerging from one another. Indeed, one of the key arguments for simulation theory and against theory theory is that rational connections lie at the heart of mental phenomena, but are not reducible to or codifiable in any set of principles of good thinking which could thus form part of a theory of mind (Heal 1995; McDowell 1998b: 325–40).

## The limits of understanding

Despite its centrality in Jaspers' conception of psychopathology and, thus, psychiatry, understanding has limits. One kind of limit is quite general and concerns its scope by contrast with natural scientific explanation. In a section of 'Causal and "meaningful" connections between life history and psychosis' called 'The limits of understanding and the universal application of explaining' he says:

> The suggestive assumption that the psychic is the area of meaningful understanding and the physical that of causal explanation is wrong. There is no real event, be it physical or of psychic nature, which is not accessible to causal explanation … The effect a psychic state may have could in principle lend itself to a causal explanation, while the psychic state itself of course must be phenomenologically (statically) understood. It is not absurd to think that it might one day be possible to have some rules which could causally explain the sequence of meaningfully connected thought processes without paying heed to the meaningful connections between them … It is therefore in principle not at all absurd to try to understand as well as to explain one and the same real psychic event. These two established connections, however, are of entirely different kinds of validity.' (Jaspers (1913) 1974: 86)

The thought here seems to be this. Understanding and explanation do not have two distinct subject matters. Rather, the difference between them is one of method or of the kind of intelligibility that they deploy. As applied in psychiatry, they share the same subject matter: 'real events' or 'thought processes', in Jaspers' terms above. These can in principle be charted in either way: either by looking to the law-like causal relations between them or by looking to the meaningful relations between them.

The idea that neutral events might be susceptible to two distinct patterns of intelligibility was recently articulated by the US philosopher of mind Donald Davidson (1917–2003). On his model of the mind, Anomalous Monism, the very same events that comprise mental events and which—according to Davidson—stand in essentially rational relations, also comprise physical events, and can be subsumed under nomological or law-like causal explanations (Davidson 1980: 207–227). When described in mental property terms, however, there are no laws that fit them. Hence—qua instantiations of mental properties—they are *anomalous*, but there are laws that fit them that use their physical or neurological properties.

Given this broad view of the relation between understanding and explanation, one might expect the following asymmetry between them. Whilst every mental event is also a physical event, not every physical event is a mental event. There were no mental properties in the event of comet Shoemaker Levy 9 colliding with Jupiter in 1994, for example. That collision was not a mental event. Thus, one might expect Jaspers to say that, whilst every event that can be understood can also be explained, not every event that can be explained can also be understood. It is rather curious, therefore, that he actually says: 'there is no event which cannot be understood as well as explained' (Jaspers (1913) 1974: 86).

Although he does not recognise that plausible general limitation on understanding—that non-mental events can only be explained not understood—Jaspers does suggest a more specific local limit in the case of psychopathology. He believes that 'primary delusions' cannot be understood. To unpack that claim, I will now outline his taxonomy of delusions.

Jaspers suggests that delusions fall into two kinds: primary and secondary or delusions proper and delusion-like ideas. Primary delusions fall into four further kinds. The first is mentioned in *General Psychopathology* almost in passing: delusional atmosphere. He says:

> with this *delusional atmosphere* we always find an 'objective something' there, even though quite vague, a something which lays the seed of objective validity and meaning ... Patients feel as if they have lost grip on things, they feel gross uncertainty ... (Jaspers 1997: 98)

To someone suffering schizophrenia, the world as a whole can seem subtly altered, uncanny, portentous or sinister. This general transformation prompts him to say elsewhere: 'We observe that a new world has come into being' (Jaspers 1997: 284). There are then three further forms of primary delusion:

> *Delusional perceptions.* These may range from an experience of some vague meaning to clear, delusional observation and express delusions of reference. (Jaspers 1997: 99)

> *Delusional ideas.* These give new colour and meaning to memory or may appear in the form of a sudden *notion*—'I could be King Ludwig's son'—which is then confirmed by a vivid memory of how when attending a parade the Kaiser rode by on his horse and looked straight at the patient. (Jaspers 1997: 103)

> *Delusional awareness.* This constitutes a frequent element particularly in florid and acute psychoses. Patients possess a knowledge of immense and universal happenings, sometimes without any trace of clear perceptual experience of them ... (Jaspers 1997: 103)

In each of these cases there is a deep change in the experience of the significance of features of the world. In the case of delusional perceptions, an experience is transformed. In the case of delusional ideas, the significance of a memory is transformed. In delusional awareness, a delusional idea springs unbidden, but in all cases, 'All primary experience of delusion is an experience of meaning' (Jaspers 1997: 103):

> [T]he *experiences of primary delusion are analogous to this seeing of meaning*, but the awareness of meaning undergoes a radical transformation. There is an immediate, intrusive knowledge of the meaning and it is this which is itself the delusional experience. (Jaspers 1997: 99)

The key feature of primary delusions, however, is that they are not understandable. Whilst secondary delusions or delusion-like ideas are, in principle, understandable in the context of a person's life history, personality, mood state or presence of other psychopathology, primary delusions have a kind of basic status:

> We can distinguish two large groups of delusion according to their *origin*: one group *emerges understandably* from preceding affects, from shattering, mortifying, guilt-provoking or other such experiences, from false perception or from the experience of derealisation in states of altered consciousness etc. The other group is for us *psychologically irreducible*; phenomenologically it is something final. We give the term '*delusion-like ideas*' to the first group; the latter we term '*delusions proper*'. (Jaspers 1997: 96)

As Andrew Sims says in a contemporary introduction to descriptive psychopathology:

> [W]hen we consider the middle aged schizophrenic spinster who believes that men unlock the door of her flat, anaesthetize her and interfere with her sexually, we find an experience that is ultimately not understandable. We can understand, on obtaining more details of the history, how her disturbance centres on sexual experience; why she should be distrustful of men; her doubts about her femininity; and her feelings of social isolation. However, the *delusion*, her absolute conviction that these things are happening to her, that they are true, is not understandable. The best we can do is to try and understand externally, without really being able to feel ourselves into her position (*genetic empathy*), what she is thinking and how she experiences it. (Sims 1988: 85)

Thus, although Jaspers places empathic understanding (both static and genetic) at the heart of psychopathology and, thus, psychiatry, he also argues that some of the key phenomena that characterise psychopathology cannot be understood. They are not understandable. If Jaspers is correct then psychiatry has a fundamental limitation, but not everybody agrees with Jaspers that key psychopathological phenomena, such as primary delusions, cannot be understood. I will now turn to some recent attempts that draw in part on philosophical models and ideas to understand, at least partially, these difficult phenomena.

## 2. **The attempt to understand psychopathology in recent philosophy of psychiatry**

In the face of the limitations on understanding suggested by Jaspers, recent philosophy of psychiatry has attempted to provide general routes for understanding psychopathological symptoms including, centrally, delusions. The aim is that philosophical analysis can provide ways of *interpreting* or *making sense* of expressions of mental disorder and thus escaping Jaspers' suggestion that 'schizophrenic psychic life' is 'ununderstandable' (Jaspers 1997: 579). There has been a great deal of recent discussion of this empathic project in philosophical psychopathology (Sass 1994; Stephens and Graham 1994; Maher 1999; Eilan 2000; Campbell 2001; Roessler 2001).

Roessler summarises (critically) one role for philosophy in much of this work thus:

> [T]he philosopher takes the part of an explorer charting certain remote regions of the 'space of reasons'. For example, John Campbell has argued that reports of thought insertion 'show that there is some structure in our ordinary notion of the ownership of a thought which we might not otherwise have suspected'. (Roessler 2001: 178)

Such a philosopher-explorer makes psychopathological phenomena understandable by showing that they are part of an, albeit enlarged, 'space of reasons' (in the phrase of the philosopher Wilfrid Sellars recently repopularised by John McDowell and Robert Brandom). They are shown to lie already within what is available to reason and hence, to some extent at least, to empathy.

Another, not incompatible, strategy discussed further below is to make sense of bizarre *beliefs* as understandable responses to bizarre pathological *experiences* (Maher 1999). We can imagine entertaining those beliefs had we had those strange experiences. Understanding psychopathological belief and experience is not a task for philosophy alone, of course, but is part of a collaborative enterprise. Chris Frith, a cognitive neurologist, for example, makes understanding at a psychological level *one* of the tasks of a cognitive neuropsychology of schizophrenia alongside neurological work:

> My approach will be to develop as complete as possible an explanation at the psychological level. In parallel with this there should eventually be a complete explanation at the physiological level. Both explanations should be continuously modified so that mapping from one to another is made easier ... (Frith 1992: 27)

The description 'at a psychological level' involves making a subject's schizophrenic mental phenomena intelligible as meaning-charged responses to the world experienced and thus potentially sharable at least through imaginative projection.

Perhaps the hardest challenge to this general empathic project are those delusions that cannot be fitted into the conventional—although widely regarded as inadequate—definition as involving 'false belief' or 'poor reality testing'. The cases I have in mind are those where there are breakdowns of the normal rational context of a belief.

Consider three kinds of case.

## Breakdowns of connections between contingent beliefs

Suppose a subject asserts—apparently at least—that they have a nuclear power station inside them, along side the assertions that they are less than 2 m tall and that nuclear power stations have a smallest dimension greater than 20 m. What are we to make of the content of their utterances or the underlying delusion? Can we say that they believe *that they have a nuclear power station inside them*? The problem is this. Such a belief content carries implications about relative sizes that are not accepted by the subject. The putative atomic content *that they have a nuclear power station inside them* clashes with the other two potential contents—about their own size and that of power stations. Thus, although the subject expresses themselves with the words 'I have a nuclear power station inside me', there is a problem in saying, from the third person stance, that they believe that they have a nuclear power station inside them. They do not believe what *we would have to believe in addition* to believe that.

## Breakdowns exemplified in *impossible* beliefs

Some psychopathological phenomena appear to involve *impossible* beliefs, for example, thought insertion or Cotard's delusion. What sense can we really attach to the sincere report that a subject is having someone else's thoughts, as in thought insertion, or the first person report that the subject is dead, as in Cotard's delusion? Both involve something more than a mere error but a severing of the conceptual connections which normally help constitute the apparent content.

## Breakdowns between beliefs and the actions they normally rationalise

A feature of some delusions is a surprising weakness in their motivational force. For example, a subject whose laboratory work is interrupted by the apparent presence of fire-breathing animals makes no attempt to alert security or the fire brigade. Sass describes this sort of case thus:

> [M]any schizophrenics who seem to be profoundly preoccupied with their delusions, and who cannot be swayed from belief in them, nevertheless treat these same beliefs with what seems a certain distance or irony ... A related feature of schizophrenic patients is what has been called their 'double bookkeeping' ... A patient who claims that the doctors and nurses are trying to torture and poison her may nevertheless happily consume the food they give her; a patient who asserts that the people around him are phantoms or automatons still interacts with them as if they were real. (Sass 1994: 21)

The underlying problem that cases of these three sorts present for an empathic understanding is that the breakdown of connections between beliefs, or between beliefs and actions, undermines grounds for the ascription of a specific content to the subject. Whilst for convenience we might say of someone that they think they are having someone else's thoughts, it is far from clear that this really is a conceivable thought, a thought *we* can ascribe to others. It appears, instead, to be brutally alien. What options are there for making sense of cases like these?

One response is to give up any attempt at empathic understanding of cases as alien as these. At the end of an article pessimistically summarising the history of the analysis of delusions as 'wrong beliefs' German E. Berrios, a psychiatrist with an academic interest in the history of psychiatry, makes the following comment:

> Delusions are likely to be empty speech acts, whose informational content refers to neither world nor self. They are not the symbolic expression of anything. Its 'content' is but a random fragment of information 'trapped' in the very moment the delusion becomes crystallized. The commonality of certain themes can be explained by the fact that informational fragments with high frequency value also have a probability of being trapped. (Berrios 1991: 12)

Rather than construing delusions as beliefs with understandable contents that suffer merely from falsity, Berrios suggests that the expression of a delusion is, strictly, empty of content, 'not the symbolic expression of *anything*'. The problem with such an approach is that does not seem to fit the clinical facts. Whilst, for reasons set out below, there are problems in taking delusions to be ordinary beliefs, it appears that they have some rational connections to some actions, beliefs and utterances.

Berrios' comment is also helpful for highlighting why a particular family of approaches to meaning or 'content' (as it is called in philosophy) seems to have greater difficulties with understanding delusions than its main rival. A useful way of drawing the distinction between approaches to meaning is to look again at the second half of the quotation above. In it, Berrios qualifies his initial radical claim (delusion as empty speech act) and goes on to suggest that the expression of a delusion may contain an *ersatz* version of content ('content'), but that this is merely a *fragment* of information, somehow *trapped* in the delusion or its expression in an utterance. What could this suggestion mean?

The easiest way to interpret it or fill it out is to adopt a 'cognitivist' or 'representationalist' approach to the content of mental states. This general approach has been championed in different ways in philosophy (Dretske 1981; Millikan 1984; Fodor 1987; Papineau 1987), in philosophy of psychiatry (Bolton and

Hill 2004), and in psychiatry by any number of cognitive neuropsychiatrists (Ellis 1996). It will be the subject of the first part of the next chapter.

A cognitive approach attempts to explain the content of mental states, and hence linguistic utterances, 'bottom up' through sub-personal processes described in information theoretic terms. Internal information-carrying states—of the brain or nervous system—are postulated which are processed by sub-personal modules. The capacity of a person as a whole to think thoughts is thus explained by the processing of internal mental representations. Of course, this raises the fundamental question: how do internal states carry meaning or representational content in the first place?

Given that the aim of this family of approaches is to *explain* intentionality, the answer to this question has to invoke something like a mechanism whose description does not presuppose any meaning-related notions. One family of approaches within philosophy elaborates the idea that a mental state means what *causes* it (to be tokened) in the brain or nervous system of a subject. Meaning is a kind of causation. If such a mechanism can be accurately described in non-question begging terms then intentionality can be shown to be an unproblematic aspect of the natural world that emerges from more basic properties. The proposed mechanisms typically have a further characteristic that is important in the context of delusions: they purport to explain how mental representations have contents independently of each other. Meaning is atomic.

With such a picture in mind it is possible to see how delusions might involve mere fragments of content as the second half of the Berrios quotation postulates. Whilst the higher level processing of mental representations corresponding to chains of thought may be faulty that need not threaten the intentionality of those basic states. There need be no *a priori* connection, on this model, between the proper functioning of the mechanisms that inject meaning into mental representations and the proper functioning of further information processing modules. There might be *epistemological* problems in discovering the fragmentary content of another person's delusion, but there is no ontological objection to the idea.

The opposed approach to the philosophy of content is 'top down'. It makes no attempt to explain how intentional content arises from neurological events described in non-intentional terms. Rather, it attempts to shed light on the place of intentional content in nature (including human nature) by describing the perspective, or stance, from which intentional states and their verbal expression 'come into view' (Wittgenstein 1953; Davidson 1984; Dennett 1987; Brandom 1994; McDowell 1998a: 171–98).

Such an approach, however, cannot easily make sense of the sort of delusions described above. The problem is that the top-down approach places a general condition on the ascription of intentional content to the 'systems' (generally *persons* except in Dennett's case) capable of entertaining it. Such ascription must presuppose a *rational* pattern in the description of mental states, utterances and behaviour. Davidson calls this the 'Constitutive Principle of Rationality' and it plays an important role in his argument that the mental cannot be reduced to or systematically mapped onto the physical. However, the central role of rationality in making sense of mental states and utterances also places limits on the possibility of articulating the content of any states which cannot be fitted into that rational pattern. The problem is that, to a first approximation, the criterion of being a thinker at all is to be interpretable according to our rational framework (Davidson 1984: 183–198). So what meaning or content can be ascribed to utterances of delusions of the sorts described above that do not fit it? Such delusions appear to violate some of the rational connections that are constitutive of thought, on this approach. (For consideration of this point see Bortolotti 2005.)

I will now outline some recent approaches to delusion. Because this is an area of the philosophy of psychiatry in flux, the examples picked are meant merely to illustrate some of the possible areas for future development. Each account varies from what might be called the proto-typical working definition of delusions which runs, roughly, as follows (based on Maher 1999):

- the individual has a belief that is false;
- this belief arises as a result of a defect of inference;
- it is held intensely and tenaciously by the individual in the face of evidence sufficient to refute it, i.e., it is "incorrigible";
- the belief is not shared by the culture of the individual in question.

## Delusions as rational responses to abnormal experiences

The US psychologist Brendan Maher has defended a model of delusion as an understandable response to an abnormal experience. In 'Anomalous Experience in Everyday Life: Its significance for psychopathology,' he suggests that there is continuity between everyday experiences of significance and those that lead to delusions (Maher 1999).

The idea is that in everyday life we can have what Maher calls 'primary feelings of significance'. Based on Jaspers' distinction between primary and secondary delusions, Maher calls these primary because they are directly experiential. They are not, for example, inferred from something else (which would make them secondary). Maher suggests that we normally refer to these by a variety of phrases such as 'feeling of awareness', 'mood', 'atmosphere', 'feeling of significance' and 'feeling of conviction'. However, the particular quality he is targeting is of an experience that something significant or important has occurred, whatever it is. Because such feelings are primary, their very existence is a basic datum for further cognitive processing, further inferences to be drawn.

One such everyday experience is that something has changed whether or not one can recognise precisely what it is. Maher gives the example of other people realising that something had changed about his (Maher's) appearance once he had shaved off a beard, but not knowing what it was and even hypothesising that it was merely a change of tie. Another such experience is the feeling of recognition, which can turn out to be mistaken. A third is a feeling of surprise. In such cases, Maher suggests, the feeling of significance can be prompted by something that is itself below the threshold of conscious experience.

Maher suggests that the same kind of phenomenon also exists within psychopathology. He gives an example from Kurt Schneider (1887–1967), a German psychiatrist who investigated schizophrenia, of a patient who reported that:

> A dog lay in wait for me as he sat on the steps of a Catholic convent. He got up on his hind legs and looked at me seriously. He saluted with his front paw as I approached him. Another man was a little way in front of me. I caught up to him hurriedly, and asked if the dog had saluted him too. An astonished 'No' told me that I had to deal with a revelation addressed to me. (Schneider 1959: 105)

Such experiences of significance are often repeated within psychopathology and from this Maher concludes:

> The fact that the experience is repeated in other contexts supports the hypothesis that its first appearance was independent of environmental input, i.e., it was endogenous. It also suggests that the spontaneous feeling of significance may become attached not only to some chance perceived feature of the external environment, but to some internal train of thought and its related imagery. It is the content of the thought that gives 'meaning' to the accidental features of the external environment. Thus the coincidence of inner thought (words and images), unrelated external stimuli, and the spontaneous biopathological activation of feelings of awareness, come together to create a seemingly instantaneous delusion. (Maher 1999: 559)

From this Maher draws his model of delusion:

1. Delusional beliefs, like normal beliefs, arise from an attempt to explain experience.
2. The processes by which deluded persons reason from experience to belief are not significantly different from the processes by which non-deluded persons do. In neither case do the beliefs typically arise from conscious application of the rules of formal logic or the principles of statistical inference.
3. Defective reasoning about actual personal normal experience is not the primary contributor to the formation of delusional beliefs. A major critical difference between delusional beliefs and non-delusional beliefs is the nature and intensity of the phenomenological experience that is being explained.

4. The origins of anomalous experience may lie in a broad band of neuropsychological anomalies. These include, but are not confined to (a) endogenous neural activation of the feeling of significance normally triggered by pre-conscious recognition of changes in a familiar environment; (b) unrecognized defects in the sensory system, such as undiagnosed hearing loss, or the endogenous activation or inhibition of the central neural representations of sensory input; (c) temporary alterations in the intensity and vividness of sensory input, as in some forms of drug intoxication; (d) neurologically based difficulties in the focusing of attention with consequent difficulty in discriminating between situationally relevant and irrelevant elements of the environment; (e) experienced discrepancies between the willed intent of a response and the actual form of the response; (f) impairment in the monitoring and calculation of recurring sequential probabilities in environmental events that is necessary to anticipate and respond effectively to later elements in the sequence. (Maher 1999: 550–1)

Or in other words:

The hypothesis proposed here is that chronology of the development of a primary delusion begins with the endogenous activation of the feeling of significance. Arising as it does from an internal neurological event that is not moderated by input from the external environment, this feeling is more intense than the normal feeling of significance. The feeling is rapidly combined with elements in the environment that are present to conscious observation at that time, plus other concurrent components of consciousness, such as ongoing trains of thought, associations to external stimuli present to observation, habitual preoccupations, and so forth. Jaspers' patient, for example, feels that suddenly things have become quite different, sees men in uniform, interprets them to be soldiers, and makes the global interpretation that there is a world war. This delusional interpretation does not terminate the feeling of significance, and the patient, noticing the scaffolding, associates it with demolition, adding the global interpretation that the town is going to be demolished. The delusional meaning comes as "given" by the combination of experience and other coincidental elements of consciousness, but it is the experience that creates the combination; it is not the delusional explanation that creates the experience. (Maher 1999: 560–1)

Maher's model has been influential. It has been developed, recently, into the so called 'two-factor model of delusion' (see below), which begins with Maher's account, but adds to it a further distortion of thinking. Unlike Maher's model, this alternative suggests that the processes by which deluded persons reason from experience to belief *are* significantly different from the processes by which non-deluded persons do. However, the starting point is the same: light can be shed on delusions by thinking of them as, in part, understandable responses to abnormal experiences. A particular attraction of Maher's model, from the point of view of empathic psychiatry, is that there is even continuity between the kind of experience that triggers delusional thinking in psychopathology and perfectly normal 'feelings of significance'.

Nevertheless, the model has two fundamental and interrelated weaknesses. On the one hand, consider the well known case that Maher also cites of the subject who, on looking at marble tables in a café, becomes convinced that the world is about to end. Maher suggests, following Jaspers himself, that, in fact, a feeling of significance *preceded* the observation of the tables and only subsequently became attached to the observation and then, presumably, was elaborated upon. Maher suggests that if the subject can find nothing in the immediate environment to explain the feeling then 'everything must have changed in some fundamental way' (Maher 1999: 560). The problem now, however, is that, whilst Maher may have shed light on the initial experience—that may be continuous with everyday cases—the adoption and maintenance of the delusion in the face of critical scrutiny becomes incomprehensible.

On the other hand, consider a case that will be discussed further in the next chapter. Chris Frith proposes an explanation of thought insertion—the delusion that one has, or that one's mind is a projection screen for, other people's thoughts—based on the breakdown of a sub-personal mechanism. Just as the brain 'signals' a distinction between changes of the visual field produced by moving one's eyes and those that result from changes in the world by labelling the former, so thoughts are also normally labelled as the product of one's own thinking. Frith suggests that, if such a labelling mechanism were to break down, one would experience one's thoughts as somehow not one's own, as alien. It is then a simple matter to ascribe them to another. 'If we found ourselves thinking without any awareness of the sense of effort that reflects central monitoring, we might well experience these thoughts as alien and, thus, being inserted' (Frith 1992: 81).

The problem in this case is not the transition from bizarre experience to rationalizing thought. It is the experience in the first place. Just what would it be to experience a thought as somehow not one's own? In this case, the problem is made worse, not better, by the everyday experience of having thoughts pop into one's mind. What could a more fundamentally alien case of a thought arising be like?

The problem takes the form of a dilemma for Maher's account. If the basic model is that of an understandable response to an abnormal experience then given the bizarre quality of the delusions in question ('best quality delusions' in Bill Fulford's phrase (Fulford 1989: 202)) two adjustments can be made to try to capture that quality. Either

- ◆ the experience is bizarre and the response to it is understandable (as in the case of thought insertion). In which case, how can we understand the experience? This is, in effect, a problem of static understanding; or

- the experience is at least continuous with normal experiences but the response to it is not (as in the case of the café tables and the end of the world). In which case, how can we understand the transition? This is, in effect, a problem of genetic understanding.

Maher's account does not seem to 'solve simultaneously for understanding and utter strangeness' in Naomi Eilan's useful metaphor (Eilan 2000: 97).

## Delusions as expressions of philosophical confusion

A more promising attempt to straddle the line between understanding and strangeness is suggested in the work of the US psychologist Louis Sass. In *The Paradoxes of Delusion* he suggests that light can be shed on the nature of schizophrenia in general—and the famous case of Paul Schreber in particular—through a comparison with the philosopher Ludwig Wittgenstein's discussion of solipsism. In broad terms, the idea is that schizophrenic experience can be modelled as an expression of a commitment to a philosophical theory. By articulating that theory and some of the motivation for adopting it, through Wittgenstein's discussion, Sass aims to make sense of Schreber's experience. He sets out his aim thus:

> In this book I attempt to do what, according to Jaspers, cannot be done: to comprehend both empathically and conceptually some of the most bizarre and mysterious symptoms of schizophrenia. (Sass 1994: 6)

More substantively he summarises his main argument as follows:

> [Schreber's] mode of experience is strikingly reminiscent of the philosophical doctrine of solipsism, according to which the whole of reality, including the external world and other persons, is but a representation appearing to a single, individual self, namely, the self of the philosopher who holds the doctrine ... Many of the details, complexities, and contradictions of Schreber's delusional world ... can be understood in the light of solipsism. (Sass 1994: 8)

The hope is thus that Schreber's experience is not simply seen as lying outside the domain of the constitutive principle of rationality:

> [Madness] is, to be sure, a self-deceiving condition, but one that is generated from within rationality itself rather than by the loss of rationality. (Sass 1994: 12)

Sass goes on to explore parallel features in Wittgenstein's discussion of solipsism and Schreber's self-narrative.

Sass' account differs in approach from that of Maher in that it postulates an overall top-down disturbance in thinking that then colours a subject's experience of the world. (Maher's account takes a basic experience, albeit not a direct experience or perception of any aspect of the world, to produce bottom- up changes in thinking.) Using a distinction made by the philosopher John Campbell, Sass' account is rationalist, rather than empiricist:

> The empiricist solution is to say that the patient is, after all, broadly rational and in command of the meaning of the words being used; it is just that we are dealing with a broadly rational reaction to some very unusual experiences … The rationalist takes the more difficult route of saying that there is a top-down disturbance in the subject's beliefs and thus faces the problem of explaining how the subject can retain a stable grasp of meaning through this disturbance. (Campbell 2001: 98)

Sass thus aims to describe that overall distortion by saying that a subject with schizophrenia has a world view in accordance with philosophical solipsism and thus he aims to make the phenomena understandable, whilst at the same time preserving their alienness. However, although the comparison is tempting, I do not believe that it is satisfactory. To argue this, I will here follow the tenor, although not the specific arguments, of the UK philosopher Rupert Read's critical response to Sass' book (Read 2001).

Read argues that there are two general Wittgensteinian reasons for thinking that Sass' invocation of Wittgenstein cannot help to make sense of Schreber. Firstly, Sass' work is an attempt to *interpret* schizophrenia, rather than *describe* it. Rather than letting Schreber's experience 'speak for itself' Sass reads significance into it, which it need not have. Read then contrasts Sass' mapping of schizophrenia onto solipsism unfavourably with the philosopher of social science Peter Winch's *rejection* of the mapping of the Azande's belief system onto Western science, rather than merely displaying its own structure (Winch 1970). The latter, he argues, is 'an example of someone—Winch—being able quite successfully 'to "follow along with" an "alien" discourse without *imposing* on it or *interpreting* it in terms other than its own' (Read 2001: 457).

There are two general Wittgensteinian reasons to be cautious of the term 'interpretation'. Wittgenstein specifically rejects a model of understanding (for example a rule, or the meaning of word) based on the interpretation of signs or symbols, whether mental or not (Wittgenstein 1953: §201). Secondly, Wittgenstein stresses our ability to hear meaning directly in speech. No work needs to be done to understand the meaning. The Wittgensteinian philosopher Stephen Mulhall argues that talk of interpretation in, for example, Donald Davidson's philosophy of content falsifies the everyday phenomenology of immediately hearing rather than having to *interpret* a sound wave (Mulhall 1990). Whether or not an accurate critique of Davidson, Mulhall correctly identifies an important aspect of our phenomenology, but it is not clear whether Sass falls foul of either of these objections. The first does not apply because Sass does not offer a general account of understanding, but whether or not the second applies depends on an ambiguity in Sass' presentation.

Whether or not Winch—and thus Read—does provide a clear distinction between interpretation and description, part of the problem in reading Sass' book is to understand precisely the kind of clarification he intends by the analogy between Schreber's schizophrenic experience and Wittgenstein's critique of solipsism. He says, for example, that 'delusional experience is *suggestive* of the world of the solipsist' (Sass 1994: 39 italics added) or is 'in perfect *accordance* with Wittgenstein's analysis of solipsism' (Sass 1994: 40 italics added). One *explicit* comments runs:

> Let us call this the attitude of 'quasi-solipsism' (since the experience is not accompanied by a full and explicit awareness in philosophical terms of the doctrine of solipsism). (Sass 1994: 39)

This leaves the weight of the qualification 'quasi' unspecified. There is a general problem here. If the commitment to solipsism were an *explicit* part of Schreber's world view then Sass' articulation could show how Schreber's utterances formed a coherent whole (although see below for a further qualification), but it would not be the original work it seems to be. Schreber's narrative would tell us of his solipsism itself. If the claim were instead that *we* can treat Schreber's utterances as following from the same sorts of motivations as philosophical solipsism, but that *Schreber* himself would not recognise this then it is not clear that we are gaining *empathic* understanding. Whilst we can find a kind of order in Schreber's account it is not the order he intends and thus we have only a kind of external structural explanation of his thought, not a shared empathic understanding. This dilemma suggests that Sass' account is a kind of unstable halfway house between understanding from within and explanation, in a more broadly causal vein, from without.

Read's second line of criticism is influenced by the recent 'resolute' interpretation of Wittgenstein's *Tractatus Logico Philosophicus* (Crary and Read 2000). The resolute reading interprets Wittgenstein's claims that the propositions contained in the *Tractatus* are nonsense literally, rather than construing them as a special sort of nonsense that points towards an ineffable truth. In other words they follow Ramsey's aphorism that 'what we can't say, we can't say and we can't whistle it either' (Ramsey 1931: 263). Read argues that the apparent sympathy towards solipsism found in the *Tractatus* is thus undercut if the whole of that work is intended as a kind of *reductio ad absurdum*. If the analogy with Wittgenstein's 'account' of solipsism is really literal nonsense then the analogy cannot provide a route to understanding or empathy as Sass intends. In fact, however, Read's idea can be assessed without taking a view on the interpretation of early Wittgenstein.

Read's account invokes a still contentious interpretation of Wittgenstein's early work. But hostility to solipsism and to a model of the mind as essentially private is a clear feature of the *later* Wittgenstein to whom Sass also appeals. Wittgenstein's arguments aim to show, not that solipsism is a coherent but false doctrine but, rather, that it does not make sense. There is thus some difficulty in construing Sass' interpretation of Schreber as providing a coherent narrative and thus a genuine way of making sense of him.

In a suggestive passage in which Sass discusses Schreber's ambivalent attitude to his delusion of having a female appearance, Sass says:

> Consider, for example, the 'specific schizophrenic incorrigibility' of what Schreber calls his 'so-called delusions'—with their absolute imperviousness to argument or external proof, and their strange, seemingly paradoxical combination of certainty with inconsequentiality. Contrary to Jaspers' views, this feature is not beyond the pale of any possible understanding. Indeed, it is natural that solipsistic claims cannot be refuted or adjudicated in any public domain. The claim that one is represented as female is not, after all, the sort of statement to which corroborative or disconfirmatory evidence could possibly be relevant. No imaginable fact—not the roughness of a beard, the narrowness of hips, or even the anatomical presence of male genitalia— could possibly refute the fact of the experience of the representing, the occurrence in a private mental space of this image of a body's femininity, this instance of seeing-as. As Wittgenstein often pointed out in his later writings ... it is nonsensical to doubt immediate subjective experience and impossible to argue (at least in any standard manner) about notions like solipsism, since normal forms of evidence are quite irrelevant to such assertions. (Sass 1994: 41)

The pairing of 'nonsensical' and 'impossible' in the last sentence of the quotation suggests that the later Wittgenstein regarded claims about subjective experience as certain and about solipsism as invulnerable to argument. Thus, it seems as though Wittgenstein provides a way of making sense of Schreber's attitude to both.

This impression is misleading. Throughout his life Wittgenstein argued that solipsism was senseless, rather than certain. Despite its initial attractions, no coherent doctrine can be arrived at. In his early notebooks he summarised his objection to solipsism in this way:

> This is the way I have travelled: Idealism singles men out from the world as unique, solipsism singles me alone out, and at last I see that I too belong with the rest of the world, and so on the one side *nothing* is left over, and on the other side, as unique, *the world*. In this way idealism leads to realism if it is strictly thought out. (Wittgenstein 1984: 85)

Solipsism is not a 'position' at all because it cannot be given a meaningful contrast with the realism to which it is supposed to be opposed. In his later *Philosophical Investigations* he argues that solipsists are best interpreted not as trying to make a claim about reality, but rather opposing a normal way of using words:

> For *this* is what disputes between Idealists, Solipsists and Realists look like. The one party attack the normal form of expression as if they were attacking a statement; the

others defend it, as if they were stating facts recognised by every reasonable human being. (Wittgenstein 1953: §402)

In addition to his opposition to solipsism, a well known aspect of the later Wittgenstein's work is his hostility to any picture of subjective experience based on essentially private inner phenomena. Thus, if Wittgenstein can be said to argue, as Sass asserts, that 'it is nonsensical to doubt immediate subjective experience' this is because it is impossible to have any attitude to subjective experience when construed as part of a 'private mental space', rather than because they are particularly certain. Neither aspect of Wittgenstein's critical discussion can provide resources for a coherent defence of and thus a way of arriving at an understanding of Schreber's views.

The novel suggestion at the heart of Sass' work is that implicit subscription to a philosophical theory—in this case solipsism—might provide a middle ground between construing schizophrenic experience as genuinely beyond understanding and as embodying a set of merely false beliefs. Philosophical theory might serve as a compromise, which can be both empathically grasped, whilst at the same time remaining intellectually alien, but whilst Wittgenstein, especially in his later work, attempted to understand the source of philosophical confusions, he did not articulate either his own or opposing philosophical ideas as coherent theses. Thus, it seems that the model cannot work.

## Delusions as framework propositions

A second use has been suggested recently for using ideas from Wittgenstein to shed light on the nature of delusions. In a paper concerned with the interpretation of the Capgras delusion, the philosopher John Campbell suggests, for further discussion at least, an analogy between delusions and Wittgenstein's *On Certainty* account of framework propositions.

> In On Certainty, Wittgenstein talked about the epistemological status of propositions like 'There are lots of objects in the world', 'The world has existed for quite a long time', 'There are some chairs and tables in this room', 'This is one hand and this is another', and so on. Wittgenstein said that beliefs expressed by such propositions are not ordinary factual beliefs, but rather form the background needed by any inquiry into truth or falsity. As he put it:

> All testing, all confirmation and disconfirmation of a hypothesis takes place already within a system. And this system is not a more or less arbitrary and doubtful point of departure for all our arguments: no, it belongs to the essence of what we call an argument. The system is not so much the point of departure, as the element in which arguments have their life. (Wittgenstein 1969: §105)

Campbell thus asks:

> In these terms, an obvious question to raise about delusions is whether the
> delusional beliefs do not have, for the subject, the epistemological status of
> Wittgenstein's framework propositions (Campbell 2001: 96).

Reporting the proposal with approval, the UK philosopher of consciousness
Naomi Eilan says:

> Our framework beliefs are those fundamental beliefs we do not question, and which
> globally constrain our inferences and our interpretation of our experiences ... The
> suggestion is that primary paranoid beliefs, such as that the IRA is out to get one,
> should be treated as constraining one's reasoning and interpretation of one's experi-
> ence in an analogous manner. They are resistant to counter-evidence because of their
> fundamental framing role ... (But contra the noise option, this does not render their
> expression senseless.) ... The main difference between this proposal and the 'strange
> experience plus rational response' proposal ... is that it focuses on a structural feature
> which could indeed capture at least one sense in which one might want to say, with
> Jaspers, that the schizophrenic's *worlds* are different. (Eilan 2000: 108–9)

Two features of framework propositions make the analogy with delusions
promising. First, framework propositions provide the context for the practice
of giving and asking for reasons that correspond to making claims of knowledge or doubt. They themselves comprise a background of certainties that are
held immune from doubt. They are not themselves known, but instead make
knowledge claims possible. By construing delusions as framework propositions, one can begin to explain their incorrigibility and the role they might
play in structuring other claims:

> [T]hey are treated as the background assumptions needed for there to be any testing
> of the correctness of propositions at all. (Campbell 2001: 96)

Secondly, unlike more traditional epistemological accounts, Wittgenstein's
picture suggests that these certainties are heterogeneous and have everyday
worldly subject matters. They are not restricted, for example, to claims about
sense data or other more familiar philosophical foundations. They can have
wider or narrower significance. Thus, the specificity of delusions is no objection to them playing just this role.

A third feature suggests the need for some care in describing the analogy.
Because framework propositions are unquestioned and lie in the background
of epistemic practices, it is difficult to describe the psychological state (if any)
that they express. It seems implausible to say, for example, that we *believe* that
'There are lots of objects in the world', 'The world has existed for quite a long
time', 'There are some chairs and tables in this room', 'This is one hand and

this is another', and so on. Such propositions seem to be more basic than any psychological attitude and instead reflect a kind of practical orientation:

> If the shopkeeper wanted to investigate each of his apples without any reason, for the sake of being certain about everything, why doesn't he have to investigate his investigation? And can one talk of belief here (I mean belief as in 'religious belief', not surmise)? All psychological terms merely distract us from the thing that really matters. (Wittgenstein 1969: §459)

Although this makes a description of the role of framework propositions a difficult task for a kind of phenomenology, it does not rule out their use in shedding light on delusions, but it does suggest that any such account must reject a definition of delusion as some form of 'wrong belief'.

Does the analogy with framework propositions help shed light on delusions? At first sight it seems that is does. The structural parallel suggests a way of coming to grips with the role of a delusion in a subject's thinking. It thus serves to shed light on how the subject could entertain a delusion in the context of evidence that would normally count against it: it is being held immune from such evidence. (Elsewhere Wittgenstein comments: "'But, if you are *certain*, isn't it that you are shutting your eyes in the face of doubt?"—They are shut.' (Wittgenstein 1953: §224).)

On reflection, however, whilst that description might give *some* sort of purchase it is not clear that it can help provide understanding that *makes sense* of the structure of the subject's world view. To get a feel for this, consider the case of 'This is one hand and this is another' taken from Moore's proof of an external world. Normally this, accompanied by a suitable demonstration, expresses a framework proposition. One can imagine contexts in which it did not serve in that role, but could be called into question, be justified and serve, instead, to express a knowledge claim. Filling out how it might be a claim either known or doubted, however, turns *not* on a general theory of how one claim might be justified or undermined by another. It turns instead on seeing in a particular, possibly hypothetical, context what justifies what. That requires that one's thinking is *sensitive* to the demands of rationality, but not that one has a *theory* of rationality.

This echoes an argument Heal provides against theory theory and in favour of simulation theory mentioned earlier as an account of knowledge of other minds (Heal 1995). Heal points out that, given the right context, virtually any false belief can be made sense of, but we are able to do this by having a mind not by having a *theory* of mind. In the case at hand, understanding how 'This is one hand' might express now a framework proposition, now a knowledge claim, depends on charting 'from within' the rational relations that support either role in different contexts.

This suggests that the understanding of the role of framework propositions manifested by Wittgenstein and shared by his readers is an understanding from *within* such a system not a theoretical stance adopted from *without*. Whilst deploying the idea of delusions as framework propositions might give a kind of external, structural description, it is not clear that we can really *make sense* of the idea of entertaining delusional contents as framework propositions even if the comparison helps codify from without some of their features. The analogy does not contribute towards empathic understanding of the nature of delusions.

## The two factor model of delusion

The two factor model of delusion has been developed by the empirically informed philosopher Martin Davies and a number of co-authors. It is based on the one factor model of Maher discussed above: delusion as an understandable response to an abnormal experience. The seminal paper: 'Monothematic Delusions: Towards a two-factor account' written by Martin Davies, Max Coltheart, Robyn Langdon and Nora Breen sets out the outlines of their contrasting, but related model as follows:

> Our proposal is that for a monothematic delusion to occur, two factors must be present. One factor is a neuropsychological anomaly with some manifestation in the experience of the subject, but this is not a sufficient condition for the occurrence of delusions. The nature of the first factor varies from delusion to delusion and from patient to patient, and … there are different kinds of neuropsychological anomalies and different kinds of unusual experiences associated with different kinds of delusion. In contrast, on the boldest version of our proposal, the nature of the second factor is the same for all deluded patients. (Davies *et al.* 2002: 147)

I will return to the nature of the second factor shortly.

The structure of the argument is elegant and simple. First, they take a set of eight kinds of delusion as test cases. These are as follows (with brief descriptions derived from their paper):

- *Capgras delusion*: 'One of my closest relatives has been replaced by an impostor.'
- *Cotard delusion*: 'I am dead.'
- *Frégoli delusion*: 'I am being followed around by people who are known to me, but who are unrecognisable because they are in disguise.'
- *Mirrored-self misidentification*: 'The person I see in the mirror is not really me.'
- *Reduplicative paramnesia*: A patient affirmed that her husband had died and was cremated four years earlier (which was true) and that her husband was a patient on the ward in the same hospital that she was in (which was

not true). She seemed to have two separate, and inconsistent, records or dossiers for her husband.

- *A delusion sometimes found in patients with unilateral neglect*: Unilateral neglect occurs in people who have had major damage to one hemisphere of the brain (almost invariably the right hemisphere). Since the right hemisphere controls the left half of the body, these patients normally have paralysed left arms and left legs. They show a marked deviation of eyes, head and trunk away from the left side of space as if they are captivated by the right side of their world. They are liable to collide with objects on their left side, they leave the food on the left half of their plates. Some patients with unilateral neglect actually deny ownership of their left arm or left hand, even when it is placed so that they have no difficulty attending to it.

- *The delusion of alien control*: 'Someone else is able to control my actions. I am a puppet and someone else is pulling the strings.'

- *Thought insertion*: 'Someone else's thoughts are being inserted into my mind.'

Next, following Maher's approach, they attempt to set out the kind of abnormal experiences that might underpin these delusions. They do this by looking to the clinical, neuropsychiatric, phenomenological and philosophical literature. They report findings that indicate that, for the first six of the eight kinds of cases, a partial explanation of the delusion is an abnormal flattening or heightening of affective responses, or from failures of monitoring. For the seventh, the delusion of alien control, they suggest an explanation in terms of the unusual experience that results from paralysis, and the loss of kinaesthetic and proprioceptive feedback from the arm. This leaves the eighth (mirrored-self misidentification): 'Does mirrored-self misidentification arise from an unusual experience of oneself as seen in a mirror?' (Davies *et al.* 2002: 142).

The abnormal experience in this case needs a little more careful articulation, but there is a kind of experiential lack that seems partially to explain it. Discussing a subject, TH, with the delusion they say:

> Before a normal subject realizes that a sheet of glass is a mirror, she may see her mirrored-self as someone just like her (but left-right reversed) in a space behind the glass, but once she learns that it is a mirror, she sees her reflected self as herself. It seems quite plausible that this difference at the level of conscious awareness is a result of the accessibility of the visuo-motor transformations, even if the subject is not actually required to do any reaching and grasping. Since the visuo-motor transformations were inaccessible for TH, it seems plausible that TH saw his reflected self as someone just like him, but not as himself. This difference from normal visual perception of mirrored-self would be a result of TH's neuropsychological anomaly. (Davies *et al.* 2002: 144)

So far, so like Maher's approach. Delusions are to be explained as understandable responses to abnormal experiences, but as Davies *et al.* go on to argue, there would be a crucial omission in any such explanation. This is highlighted by a predictive failure of Maher's model:

> On Maher's view, simply suffering from any one of these experiences would be sufficient to produce a delusion, because a delusion is the normal response to such unusual experiences. It follows that anyone who has suffered neuropsychological damage that reduces the affective response to faces should exhibit the Capgras delusion; anyone with a right hemisphere lesion that paralyzes the left limbs and leaves the subject with a sense that the limbs are alien should deny ownership of the limbs; anyone with a loss of the ability to interact fluently with mirrors should exhibit mirrored-self misidentification, and so on. However, these predictions from Maher's theory are clearly falsified by examples from the neuropsychological literature. (Davies *et al.* 2002: 144)

Davies and his co-authors point out that, in at least some of the test cases, subjects can have the unusual experiences without developing the corresponding delusions. The abnormal experience is not *sufficient* for developing the delusion. Thus, for example, patients with depersonalization disorder may say that it is *as if* an alien were controlling their actions. The DSM definition of depersonalization disorder describes feelings 'like an automaton' and 'a sensation of lacking control of (his or her) actions'. Crucially, however, such a subject 'maintains intact reality testing (e.g., awareness that it is only a feeling and that he or she is not really an automaton)' (American Psychiatric Association 1994: 500–2). From this, it follows that the *experience* of alien control is not sufficient for full blown *delusion*.

They conclude:

> It is the second factor that explains the difference between a mirrored-self misidentification patient such as TH and a patient with mirror agnosia or between a patient with the alien control delusion and a patient with alien control experiences as part of depersonalization disorder ...
>
> The argument for a second factor is, of course, strengthened if we can find other examples of non-delusional subjects who have neuropsychological anomalies and consequent unusual experiences. Indeed, the ideal situation would be to have non-delusional cases corresponding to each of the eight delusions in our battery. There is more work to be done here. We do not know of any such non-delusional cases that correspond to the Frégoli delusion, to reduplicative paramnesia, or to thought insertion, but in our view, based on the examples of non-delusional patients that we have mentioned in this section, the argument for the two-factor proposal is already strong. (Davies *et al.* 2002: 147)

Of course, it is one thing to point out that the kind of experience deployed in Maher's one factor model is insufficient to explain delusion; it is another to pinpoint the second factor in each case. It may be that the additional factors needed to turn a necessary element—the abnormal experience—into a sufficient explanation vary from case to case, whether individual subjects or types of delusion. However, Davies and his co-authors at least discuss the possibility that there might be just one kind of additional factor, which has to do with a subject's failure to reject the bizarre nature of the delusional content.

They consider two possible routes from unusual experience to delusional belief:

> On the first route, delusional patients are aware that there is something unusual or anomalous about their experience, and they construct an explanation for the occurrence of this unusual feature. On the second route, delusional patients simply believe what they perceive; they implicitly assume that perception is veridical. (Davies *et al.* 2002: 150)

On the second route, the delusional content is already part of how the world seems to them. Thus, in the case of Capgras, the perceptual experience would have the content: this is someone who looks like my relative, but is not really him/her. On the first route, the experience is more modest. There is a perception of someone who looks like a relative and there is also an absence of a sense of familiarity, but the claim that the person is an impostor is a further conclusion devised to explain the visual experience combined with the feeling.

As the authors go on to discuss, neither route offers a clear explanation as to why subjects suffer quite specific or 'monothematic' delusions or how some are able to recognise that their delusions are implausible. If, for example, one postulates general cognitive deficits to explain, on route one, why a bizarre explanatory hypothesis is not rejected on the basis of further first person experience, stored knowledge or testimony from other people, then why do subjects of such delusions not have many other bizarre beliefs, and how can they sometimes recognise their delusion to be implausible? If, on the second route, one tries to explain why deluded subjects do not reject the bizarre content of a complex experience, it seems likely that they should also be prey to many visual illusions. Thus, although Davies speculates that the second factor has something to do with failure to reject a bizarre belief, he admits it is difficult to explain just what this factor might actually be:

> The second factor in the aetiology of delusions can be described superficially as the loss of the ability to reject a candidate for belief on the grounds of its implausibility and its inconsistency with everything else that the patient knows. However, in the final section we pointed out two problems that confront any attempt to say more about the nature of this second factor ... At present, we do not know how those problems are to be solved, but our provisional view is that we do better to assume the second route from unusual experience to delusional belief and then to conceptualize the second factor as a failure to inhibit a pre-potent doxastic response. (Davies *et al.* 2002: 153–4)

The key objection to the two factor model is, however, the same as for Maher's original bizarre experience plus rational response. Adding the second factor does not address the fact that the original abnormal experience remains incomprehensible, but now, in addition, the second factor also looks problematic. What sense can we make of not rejecting such implausible explanatory theories? Whatever predictive success the two factor model might enjoy it seems to fail as a route to empathic understanding of psychopathology.

## Delusions seen from an engaged rather than estranged perspective

The final approach to delusion I will outline takes a different tack. Starting with a distinction between approaches to delusion that focus on a fault in inferential reasoning and those like Maher's that start with abnormal experiences to which there is a rational response (a distinction that roughly maps onto rationalist and empiricist in Campbell's terms), the UK philosopher of psychiatry Richard Gipps (writing with Bill Fulford) argues that there is a third fundamentally distinct option, which deconstructs that distinction.

Gipps argues that the separation of experience and inference is a sign of an 'estranged epistemology', which resembles cognitivist approaches to meaning (discussed in Chapter 4 below). The estranged conception explains intentionality through internal states and these are connected to the world, or animated, though experiences. (In cognitivism, the mediation is through causation.) On the estranged conception:

> My understanding and knowledge of the world are products of reflection on my experience, which precedes such reflection. That I may be completely unaware of any such reflection is supposedly not to the point; the cognitive processes, which mediate from perceptual input to comprehension of what is seen are typically near automatic and running completely outside of conscious awareness. (Gipps and Fulford 2004: 229–230)

Gipps also suggests that the estranged conception characterises the subject as a detached contemplator. This point corresponds to the German phenomenologist Martin Heidegger's (1889–1976) criticism of Descartes. Heidegger argues that, on Descartes' account, subjects' basic understanding of the world is based on detached contemplation of bare objects, which are 'present at hand'. By contrast Heidegger stresses the role of a practical engagement with objects taken to be 'handy tools' or 'ready to hand' (Heidegger 1962). This practical relation grounds intentionality or the 'aboutness' of thoughts—the 'practical turn' is also found in the later Wittgenstein's work. Similarly, Gipps argues that there is a more basic practical relation to the world that is revealed in an 'engaged' model of epistemology or intentionality.

With this characterisation in place, Gipps also makes a further claim that runs counter to an estranged conception. Experience is not a neutral starting point that can later be taken up into this or that understanding of the world. It is not a kind of uncomprehending 'given', which must always be further worked over by thought. Rather, it itself is the locus of our foundational grasp, which is typically active and engaged, rather than reflective and disengaged:

> Perception is not a matter of sensory 'input' to an inner mind; rather it is a natural comprehending relation of people (and not of minds) to the world around them. Experience on this view is not typically a *precursor* of understanding, but itself one of the media of our comprehension. (Gipps and Fulford 2004: 230)

Again, there are philosophical resources to support this view. The philosopher John McDowell, building on the criticism of the 'Myth of the Given' voiced by Wilfrid Sellars, argues that experience is always already conceptualised (Sellars 1997; McDowell 1994). All seeing is 'seeing as', and philosophers such as Alva Noë (2004) and Susan Hurley (1998) have argued that our experience is also intrinsically agential.

On the engaged conception, the choice between either faulty inferences or abnormal experiences is a false choice. Both stand or, as in the case of delusions, fall together:

> On the engaged conception delusions are not to be understood as a rational attempt by the understanding *to make sense of abnormal experience*, but rather as a failure *in* experience *to make sense of the world*. Such a failure in experience is not a matter of seeing *things* that are not there (hallucination or illusion), but rather of experiencing *meaning* which is either not there at all or which is experienced in a distorted, skewed, form. The failure, then, is not in the bringing to bear of the understanding on experience, nor in the experience being presented to the understanding, but a failure in that understanding contained *within* our experience of the world. The engaged conception allows us to dismount from the seesaw of delusion as a failure in reason or experience by viewing delusion as a failure in our primary experiential encounter with the world, which is already a comprehending of it. (Gipps and Fulford 2004: 233)

Whilst Gipps and Fulford aim to shed light on delusion, it is not clear that they aim to help empathic understanding. On their account, there is a fundamental pre-reflexive relation between subjects and the world which can be distorted or fragmented. When it is, both experiences of the world and also the general structure of a world view are distorted. Thus factoring out elements to explain delusions will fail. But at the same time, this failure of basic intentionality also precludes making sense of the content of delusions. The engaged epistemology is part of an account of what makes thought possible and thus suggests what might be undermined in psychopathology. But this is not to say that an engaged epistemological stance provides a route to understanding psychopathology.

## 3. **Conclusions**

Jaspers emphasises the role of understanding within psychopathology and thus psychiatry to balance the role of causal, nomological explanation. Thus, his picture of psychiatry combines aspects of the 'space of reasons' as well as the 'realm of law'. However, he also argues that central aspects of psychopathology—primary delusions—cannot be understood. They are, on the one hand, mental, rather than merely brutally causal phenomena, but on the other hand, they cannot be grasped through the paradigmatic method of making sense of mental phenomena.

Recent models within the philosophy of psychiatry have attempted to display the logic of delusions in such a way that they can be at least partially understood. The models attempt, that is, to 'solve simultaneously for understanding and utter strangeness', but as I have argued, although they suggest a number of interesting promising partial parallels between the nature of delusions and philosophical accounts, none so far looks to be able to provide a route to understanding.

Perhaps that is unsurprising. Maybe the problem is that a condition of adequacy of an interpretative approach is that it should depict the utter strangeness of at least some central psychopathological phenomena and that is an impossible task. Interpreting or understanding but still finding utter strangeness are incompatible goals.

If so, then perhaps the work of the Italian psychiatrist and phenomenologist Giovanni Stanghellini embodies the best approach. In his book of essays *Disembodied Spirits and Deanimated Bodies* (Stanghellini 2004), he treads a middle ground between an external characterisation of schizophrenia and an interpretative task. Thus, on the one hand, he suggests that schizophrenia can be seen as a breakdown of three distinct areas:

- the ability to synthesise different senses into a coherent perspective on the world (coenesthia);
- the ability to share a common world view with other members of a community (*sensus communis*);
- a basic pre-intellectual grasp of, or attunement to, social relations (attunement).

Stanghellini says: 'The philosophical kernel of my proposal is to show how all these dimensions of the phenomenon of common sense (coenesthia, *sensus communis*, and attunement) *are related to each other*' (Stanghellini 2004: 10).

Although the first element here has not been mentioned in this chapter, it broadly fits Maher's abnormal experience model. The second aspect resembles Campbell's and Eilan's invocations of a breakdown in Wittgensteinian framework propositions and the third is akin to the practical turn in Gipps' engaged epistemology. However, Stanghellini does not attempt to use these ideas to step wholeheartedly inside the world view of subjects with schizophrenia. Rather breakdowns of these are postulated as clues to interpret the strange things that sufferers report, but a basic phenomenon remains: the inaccessibility of experiences and thoughts:

> Listening to a person affected by schizophrenia is a puzzling experience for more than one reason. If I let his words actualize in me the experiences he reports, instead of merely taking them as symptoms of an illness, the rock of certainties on which my life is based may be shaken in its most fundamental features. The sense of being *me* the one who is now seeing this sheet, reading these lines and turning this page; the experience of perceptual unity between my seeing this book, touching its cover and smelling the scent of freshly printed pages; the feeling that it is me the one who agrees or disagrees with what I am reading; the sense of belonging to a community of people, of being attuned to the others and involved in my actions and future; the taken-for-granted of all these doubtless features of everyday life, may be put at jeopardy. Although my efforts to understand, by suspending all clinical judgement, allow me to see these person's self-reports as a possible configuration of human consciousness, I must admit that there is something incomprehensible and almost inhuman in these experiences, something that makes me feel radically different from the person I am listening to. (Stanghellini 2004: 111)

This suggests that understanding is an ongoing but sometimes ultimately impossible task. The clinician has to make a series of interpretative judgements taking broad account of the life of the sufferer from, for example, schizophrenia. Such judgements can help towards at least a partial understanding of the person as a whole, whilst at the same time taking account of the vividly alien quality of their psychopathological experiences.

On this approach, interpretative judgements presuppose that, as it were, the basic unit of meaning is the life of the whole person. Attempts at individual interpretation of specific delusions can be guided by a more general framework that takes schizophrenia, for example, to involve a breakdown of common sense (Stanghellini), or which begins its account of meaning from an engaged perspective and thus takes experience to depend on a shared basic understanding of the world (Gipps). However, those tools only go so far and, once they have given out, the interpretation of individual experiences has to be replaced—as Gipps and Stanghellini imply—by a sometimes partial and shifting understanding of the person as a whole based on contextual judgements. As in other areas of psychiatry, there is no quick route to bypass the need for good and sensitive judgement.

## Chapter 4

# Theorising about meaning for mental health care

## Plan of the chapter

As Chapter 3 described, a central aim of psychiatry is to understand the meanings and significance of subjects' experiences no less than to explain the aetiology of mental illness. Psychiatry thus, in Jaspers' terms, trades in reasons as well as causes; in fact, because it seems likely that reasons are a sub-species of causes—reasons can cause actions or cause other reasons to be believed—it is better to say, in the terms repopularised by the philosopher John McDowell (following Wilfrid Sellars), that psychiatry charts both the 'space of reasons' as well as the 'realm of law' (McDowell 1994).

Whilst Chapter 3 examined the limits of understanding, this chapter concerns another fundamental matter for psychiatry: the place of meaning in nature. It concerns, in other words, the relationship between understanding meaning and explaining through scientific laws. What account can be given of meanings (both the meaning of utterance and also the meaning or, as it is more usually expressed, the content of mental states)? The ontological question about what sorts of things meanings are sheds light on the methodological question (raised in Chapter 3) about the relationship of understanding and explanation.

The question of the relation of reasons and causes, or better of the space of reasons and the realm of law, is a central question in the philosophy of mind. The 'mind–body' problem centres on how mind and matter, or mental and physical properties, are related. This chapter concerns an aspect of that problem: how meaning or intentionality (the philosophical word for the way thoughts or sentences can be *about* something) or the semantic aspect of mental states is related to other non-meaningful, non-intentional, non-semantic aspects of the world. One challenge is thus to naturalise meaning, much as Chapter 1 considered how to naturalise the concept of mental illness. That is, the challenge is to shed light on meaning by showing how it can be unproblematically part of nature. There are two main sections covering the two most influential approaches to meaning taken in mental health care: cognitivism in psychiatry and discursive psychology. A third section looks at the positive lessons that can be drawn from Wittgenstein's work including critically examining Derek Bolton and Jonathan Hill's *Mind, Meaning and Mental Disorder* (Bolton and Hill 2004).

The first part of the chapter examines the approach to meaning, found in cognitivist psychology and psychiatry, according to which meanings are carried by internal information carrying states of the brain. The second part contrasts this with social constructionist discursive psychology. I will argue that both are flawed accounts of the meaning or content of mental states. Meaning can neither be reduced to states in the head nor to ongoing production in conversations. In a third section, drawing on the work of the philosopher Wittgenstein, I will argue that both linguistic meaning and mental content are irreducible aspects of the natural world, but this being so psychiatry has to recognise a broader conception of nature than is held by many. The world does not just contain features that could, in principle, be described by a completed physics. It also contains meanings. (In Chapter 5, building on the arguments of Chapters 1 and 2, I will argue that it contains values.)

## 1. **Cognitivism, the mind and inner states**

Cognitivism is a family of approaches to the mind that treats the mind on the model of an information processing computer. Computational theories of mind are in this broad sense cognitivist. This connection is expressed in standard textbooks of cognitive psychology. In his *Explorations in Cognitive Neuropsychology*, Parkin says:

> Cognitive psychology can be defined as the branch of psychology which attempts to provide scientific explanation of how the brain carries out complex mental functions such as vision, memory, language and thinking. Cognitive psychology arose at a time when computers were beginning to make a major impact on science and it was

perhaps natural that cognitive psychologists should draw an analogy between computers and the human brain. The computer analogy was used frequently to draw up a model of the brain in which mental activity was characterised in terms of the flow of information between different stores. (Parkin 1996: 3)

A key element of this approach is that for information (or content) to be processed there have to be bearers of that information (or content). Thus, the mind or brain is populated with states or 'representations' that carry meaning or *encode* content (for the latter phrase see (Bolton and Hill 2004)). In other words, a computational approach to the mind presupposes a medium of computation: a system of inner states or representations. For this reason, in philosophy, this approach is more usually called 'representationalism'.

Perhaps the most explicit formulation of this approach within *philosophy* is provided by the work of the US philosopher Jerry Fodor. Spelling out the explanatory burden of the comparison with computers, he comments:

> Real computers characteristically use at least two different languages: an input/output language in which they communicate with their environment and a machine language in which they talk to themselves (i.e. in which they run their computations). 'Compilers' mediate between the two languages … My point is that, though the machine must have a compiler if it is to use the input/output language, it doesn't *also* need a compiler for the machine language. What avoids an infinite regression of compilers is the fact that the machine is *built* to use the machine language … The critical property of the machine language is that its formulae can be paired directly with the computationally relevant physical states of the machine in such a fashion that the operations the machine performs respect the semantic constraints on formulae in the machine code. (Fodor 1975: 65–7)

Computers are designed in such a way that their inner physical states have causal properties, which mirror the computational significance of the contents that those states encode. Thus, the rules that govern the syntax of elements within machine language are matched to physical laws, which govern the causal properties of the states that encode those elements. (Fodor talks of semantic, rather than syntactic constraints. I will return to that more ambitious claim shortly.)

With the general metaphor in place, and in particular the idea that a computational approach requires a medium of computation or set of representations, Fodor summarises the key idea behind representationalism (and, I suggest, cognitivism) thus:

> At the heart of the theory is the postulation of a language of thought: an infinite set of 'mental representations' which function both as the immediate objects of propositional attitudes and as the domains of mental processes. More precisely, RTM [the Representationalist Theory of Mind] is the conjunction of two claims:
>
> *Claim 1* (the nature of propositional attitudes): For any organism O, and any attitude A toward the proposition P, there is a ('computational'/'functional') relation R and a mental representation MP such that MP means that P, and O has A iff O bears R to MP

> *Claim 2* (the nature of mental processes): Mental processes are causal sequences of tokenings of mental representations. (Fodor 1987: 16–17)

Claim 2 emphasises the materialist stance of the project. Since mental processes are causal sequences of mental representations, the latter are the sorts of states that can stand in causal relations, that is, they have physical properties. They are internal states like the electronic states of computers. Mental representations are really states of the brain or nervous system.

Claim 1 spells out an information processing or cognitivist approach to content-laden mental states or propositional attitudes. If Smith hopes that it will rain then we can say, albeit a little unnaturally, that she has an attitude of hoping to the proposition: *it will rain*. Fodor explains this by saying that she has a mental representation that means or encodes the content *it will rain*, and that Smith has the kind of computational or functional relation to that mental representation which corresponds to *hoping*. This latter suggestion flows from the attractive idea that we do different things with, for example, our hopes and our fears. We attempt to bring about whatever we hope for and try to avoid what we fear. So representations placed in what is sometimes metaphorically called a 'hope box' play a different functional role in our thinking from those placed in a 'fear box'. However, Claim 1 also makes plain the idea that representationalism requires an account of how a representation that is a state of the brain or nervous system can *encode* its content.

In order to point to the challenge that this approach faces I will look briefly at a short discussion in a textbook (Andrew Ellis' *Human Cognitive Neuropsychology*). The key point is that the challenge is ignored in this, as in many other, text books. In fact, this book is commendable and rare in even making the limited comments it does. Given that such books summarise the central shared assumptions of a discipline, this absence is significant.

At the start of a chapter called 'Recognising and understanding spoken words', Ellis sets out the information processing assumptions, which characterise the approach he takes to the area:

> Spoken language travels from speaker to hearer as a sound wave. That sound wave is an extremely rich source of information … There is of course linguistic information encoded in the speech wave … We shall … principally be concerned with recognising spoken words and extracting their meaning … (Ellis 1996: 143)

Deficit studies suggest that there are different abilities in play in different exercises including repeating nonsense words, repeating words of a language, repeating or responding in another way (e.g. giving antonyms) to words whose meaning is known. This fact, in turn, suggests that there might be different 'routes' between different, but related mental modules that perform different functions. Such relations are represented in the familiar 'functional dependence' diagrams that play an important role in cognitive psychology. In these diagrams, information is represented as passing from one module to another along specific hypothesised routes. Ellis gives a simple example (Figure 4.1).

He gives the following interpretation of this diagram:

> [The figure] provides three 'routes' between hearing a word and saying it. The first route is through word meanings and the two lexicons; the second is provided by the direct link between the auditory analysis system and the phoneme level; and the third is provided by the arrow linking the auditory input lexicon to the speech output lexicon. This would allow heard words to activate their entries in the speech output lexicons directly, without going via the representations of word meanings in the semantic system. (Ellis 1996: 144)

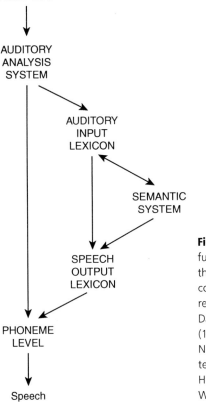

**Figure 4.1** Simple functional model for the recognition, comprehension, and repetition of spoken words. Data from Ellis, A. W. (1996) Human Cognitive Neuropsychology: a textbook with readings, Hove: Psychology Press. With permission.

The second and third routes are described thus:

> One way to repeat a heard word would be to activate its entry in the speech output lexicon, release the phonemic form, and articulate it. This would be to take a route straight through … [the figure]. However, normal people can also repeat aloud unfamiliar words or non-words like 'fep' or 'flootil', for which there will be no entry in either the auditory input lexicon or the speech output lexicon. In … (the figure) therefore we need a bypass route from the acoustic analysis system, to the phoneme level. The bypass route *must* be used to repeat unfamiliar words or non words. It *could* be used for real words (treating them as if they were non-words), but real words can also be repeated via the input and output lexicons. (Ellis 1996: 144)

So far so good, but in a chapter called 'Recognising and *understanding* spoken words' (italics added) we might also reasonably expect that a cognitivist treatment would be given, not just to routes, which correspond to *bypassing* an understanding of the meaning of words, but also to routes that *involve* understanding meaning. Ellis, however, provides only one description of the working of the semantic system here. The route that involves it is described thus:

> We propose in [the figure] … that the first stage of auditory word recognition performed by an early auditory analysis system attempts to identify phonemes in the speech wave. The results of this analysis are transmitted to the auditory input lexicon where a match is sought against the stored characteristics of known words. If the match is a good one, the appropriate recognition unit in the auditory input lexicon will be activated. It, in turn, will then activate the *representation of the meaning of the heard word in the semantic system* … (Ellis 1996: 144 italics added)

The striking omission is any further characterisation of *how* the semantic system processes the representations of meanings of words. One possible reason that this is not taken to be worth developing is that representing the meaning of a word can be thought to be a straightforward matter. The word itself can be used to represent its meaning. (Just as one can say 'rouge' in French means red, so one can also say 'red' means red.) However, that clearly will not do in this context in which the semantic system pairs words with their meanings.

There are, furthermore, serious difficulties to be overcome in this area. Consider, for example, what might stand as the representation of the meaning of a simple signpost such as a pointing arrow. If one understands the sign—if one has grasped its meaning—then one understands which way it points. It points towards, rather than away from, the arrowhead. So, schematically, one might attempt to represent that meaning in the semantic system of someone who has understood the signpost with a pointing arrow, pointing in the same direction as the signpost's arrow. That mental representation will however only represent pointing in the direction of the arrowhead if one already understands how to interpret it. The problem is that specifying the correct interpretation of the inner representation—through another representation—would generate a vicious regress.

This point is familiar from Wittgenstein and his interpreters, some of whom have taken it to cast doubt on the very idea that we can mean anything by a word (Wittgenstein 1953; Kripke 1982; Wright 1991). Nevertheless, the sceptical force of this line of thought can be constrained by noting that it stems from an assumption that is not obligatory: that meaning has to be theorised about by postulating a medium of representations within 'inner space' to bear or encode the content of mental states (including understanding the meaning of a word). Such states stand in inner space like signposts in need of interpretation. The assumption that meaning is to be explained in this way is, however, an assumption that underpins a cognitivist account of mind. (I will discuss this assumption, and the connection between scepticism about meaning, constructionism and Wittgenstein in the second half of this chapter.)

The objection that representationalism owes an account of how inner states can encode meanings or contents is one with which representationalist *philosophers* are familiar. It is an area, therefore, where co-operation between philosophers and cognitive psychologists and psychiatrists might be fruitful. The general strategy taken by such philosophers is to combine talk of inner states and their causal relations with one another (see Fodor's Claim 2 above) with causal relations between those inner states and the items in the world they are supposed to represent. In Jaspers' terminology, it is to show how causes can give rise to reasons. More recently, it is called a causal theory of reference. In virtue of being *caused* (or 'caused to be tokened') by worldly items, inner states represent them.

This approach is still a live research programme within the philosophy of thought, but it is fair to say that all the proposals so far put forward about how to characterise the right sort of relation between an inner state and a worldly item so as to explain the content that the former encodes *without begging the question* have met substantial criticism.

One major challenge recognised by philosophers who advocate a causal theory of reference is to show how false thought is possible. Suppose that on a dark night a subject mistakenly takes the outline of a plump horse to be a cow. If so, the horse causes the subject to have a cow-thought, the same kind of thought that the subject would have on looking at a cow in good observing conditions, albeit mistakenly on this dark occasion. However, the danger for a causal theory of reference is that, according to its basic tenets, the thought means or, more precisely, has the content that corresponds to what causes it. Thus, the subject's thought means, or has the content, 'cow or plump horse seen at night', but if so, contrary to the original description, the subject has not had a false thought that there is a cow, but a true thought that there is a cow *or* a plump horse seen at night. The challenge to a purely causal account such as Fodor's is to prevent it collapsing into an account where *whatever* causes an inner state constitutes its content. That would lead to the content of the inner state being a disjunction of all its possible causes, thus banishing the possibility that one could ever think a false thought. The problem of accounting for false thought is thus often called the 'disjunction problem'.

Fodor's preferred solution to the disjunction problem is elegant and minimal. It is to distinguish between causal connections which are constitutive of content and those which are not, in terms of asymmetric dependence (Fodor 1987). A type of mental representation has the content 'cow' if cows cause it to be tokened in the 'belief box' of a thinker and if those occasions on which it is caused by non-cows depend asymmetrically on the connection to cows. (Thus, if the former connection had not existed—because the mental representation had a different content or there were no cows—then the latter would not have existed either, but not vice versa.) Occasions when non-cows cause the 'cow' mental representation to be tokened can now be counted as errors.

Fodor's proposal has received much critical attention. There have been many articles published which attempt to show that Fodor's theory gives the wrong result in particular circumstances (e.g. Loewer and Rey 1991). However, there is another more general problem highlighted by Godfrey-Smith (Godfrey-Smith 1989). He asks what resources a *purely causal* theory has for distinguishing between the independent causal relation that determines the content of a mental representation and those dependent causal relations that correspond to error?

Consider a mental representation that is caused by normal-looking horses, athletic cows, muddy zebras and so forth. One obvious interpretation of this is that the representation encodes horse-thoughts, and that the connections between it and some cows and zebras asymmetrically depends on the connection to horses. But there is another interpretation that is equally plausible, given only the facts about causal connections. That is that the mental representation encodes a disjunctive content including normal-looking horses, some cows and zebras. There is, after all, a *reliable* causal connection between those animals and the representation. It is only *given* the content of the mental representation that one can determine which connections are fundamental and which are dependent, which would hold in nearby possible worlds and which would not. What this suggests is not just that there is a problem with Fodor's particular solution, but that there is something generally wrong with attempts to reduce intentional notions to purely causal ones. Something is omitted by the causal account. It cannot determine which the *correct* application is.

An alternative strategy is to invoke an evolutionary biological account to put further constraints on a causal account. Very roughly, an inner state encodes those contents that best explain its biological utility. The most influential proponent of this approach is the philosopher Ruth Garrett Millikan (Millikan 1984, 1995). She argues that the distinction between correctness and incorrectness in the tokening of a mental representation can be defined by reference to its functioning in accord with its biological function.

It is worth noting first just how ambitious this version of the reductionist project is. It is not merely the claim that a general evolutionary theoretical explanation can be given for the possession of intentional mental states (of why it is advantageous to be able to represent the world). It is rather that each particular type of content can be explained in this way. Furthermore, the explanations cannot be question-begging: the selective advantages conferred must be characterisable in non-intentional terms. The meaning must drop out of the evolutionary theory.

A teleological account of function is, however, a form of *interpretational* theory in the sense that the characterisation of the function which explains the survival of a trait is, in effect, an interpretation of the past behaviour. Past behaviour replaces inner states as the set of signs that has to be interpreted, but there is no limit to the different ways past behaviour can be interpreted. Like the interpretation of signs, such behaviour is *consistent* with an unlimited number of possible functions or rules including both continuations that seem natural and logical, and an unlimited number of other 'bent' rules that deviate in unnatural ways. What ensures the determinacy of biological function— what selects just one of the rules—is an explanation of the presence of a trait couched in intentional terms which interprets what the trait is for. However, finite past behaviour can be explained as exemplifying many different or 'bent' functions or rules, all of which would have been equally successful in the past, but which diverge in the future. (For the terminology 'bent rule', see Blackburn 1984 and discussion in the second half of this chapter.)

Millikan herself dismisses these possible alternatives by stressing the claim that the explanation of a trait turns on what caused it to survive *in the past*. She considers the case of the rules which govern a hoverfly's mating behaviour. Such flies are disposed to take flight in a particular direction depending on the angle at which a potential mate is observed. Engineering limitations, however, mean that if the mate arrives in the blind spot of the fly, it takes no action. Nevertheless, the biological *function* of the (relevant trait of the) fly is to take off at an angle that is a regular trigonometric function of the observed mate's initial position. Proper function and disposition do not coincide for all angles but the correct function can nevertheless be identified. She argues:

> [The 'bent' rule] is not a rule the hoverfly has a biological purpose to follow. For it is not because their behaviour coincided with *that* rule that the hoverfly's ancestors managed to catch females, and hence to proliferate. In saying that, I don't have any

> particular theory of the nature of explanation up my sleeve. But surely, on any reasonable account, a complexity that can simply be dropped from the explanans without affecting the tightness of the relation of explanans to explanandum is not a *functioning* part of the explanation. (Millikan 1993: 221)

The claim is that 'bent' rules introduce additional and unnecessary complexities, which can be dispensed with without damaging the explanation of the success of a biological trait. The problem with this reply is that it works only in the context in which the simplicity of an explanation can be assessed in a non-question-begging way. The problem is that the explanation of the survival value of the trait corresponding to a particular mental content has to be given without presupposing its content. Recall that the articulation of a proper function is not a matter of looking to behavioural dispositions, but selecting from that causal history a function that best explains it, and now the question is what governs the pattern of this kind of explanation?

The problem is that that pattern is visible only to someone sensitive to the structure of the space of reasons not just the realm of natural law. The latter might be able in principle to explain the detailed history of a trait, but not identify its function nor, thus, its *successes* and *failures*. Such a determination, however, is an exemplification of the structure of the space of reasons, not an independent explanation of it. (This criticism mirrors the criticism in Chapter 1 of Wakefield's partial reduction of illness via biological function.)

There are other difficulties of detail to be overcome if this general approach is to be successful, but I want to mention one other general problem. It is set out in a paper by the Wittgensteinian philosopher John McDowell. He characterises the dual role of representationalist or cognitivist accounts of the meaning of inner states thus:

> Representational bearing on the external world figures in a mode of description of those states and events that takes into account not only their intrinsic nature but also their relations to the outside world. Light enters into the picture, so to speak, only when we widen our field of view so as to take in more simply the layout of the interior ... What makes this unsatisfying, however, is the way in which the internal component of the composite picture, and not the compositely conceived whole, irresistibly attracts the attributes that intuitively characterise the domain of subjectivity ... Quite generally, nothing could be recognisable as a characterisation of the domain of subjectivity if it did not accord a special status to the perspective of the subject. But we create the appearance of introducing light into the composite picture precisely by allowing that picture to take in all kinds of facts that are not conceived in terms of the subject's point of view. So if the composite picture contains anything corresponding to the intuitive notion of the domain of subjectivity, it is the dark interior. The difficulty is palpable: how can we be expected to acknowledge that our subjective way of being in the world is properly captured by this picture, when it portrays the domain of our subjectivity—our cognitive world—in such a way that, considered from its own point

of view, that world has to be considered as letting in no light from outside? (McDowell 1998a: 250–1)

This passage suggests that even if it were possible to solve the disjunction problem—at least to the extent of providing a distinction in non-question-begging terms of those causes of the tokening of inner states which correspond to their content and those which do not—a problem would remain. The problem is that the subject described by a cognitivist account appears to be out of touch with, alienated or estranged from—to use Gipps' term introduced in Chapter 3—the world. Even the mental state that corresponds to opening one's eyes to and experiencing the world is construed as a free-standing state in inner space connected to the outer world only by causal relations, but how can such a state be *about* anything? How can such inner states be anything but blind? The general explanatory picture at work here seems not to contain the right sort of materials to explain how thought and experience is able to bear on the world at all.

As McDowell goes on to suggest, although modern cognitivist approaches to the mind shun Descartes' view that it is a kind of immaterial substance, they share a similar strategic assumption. The mind is populated with states which could be fully described without mentioning their relation to the world. The motivation—common to Cartesianism and cognitivism—is that only so can there be a *science* of mental states, but once the idea of the mind as 'inner space' is taken literally its bearing on the outer world becomes mysterious.

In this subsection I have described a general problem for any cognitivist account of mental states as free-standing inner representations. In the next subsection I wish to suggest that the assumption that the states are independent, not only of the world but of their subjects, is also a cause for concern. I will do this by considering a cognitivist account of the psychopathological phenomenon thought insertion.

## A cognitivist account of thought insertion

In thought insertion, subjects have the delusion that their thoughts are somehow not their own:

> In thought insertion, [a subject] experiences thoughts that do not have the feeling of familiarity, of being his own, but he feels that they have been put in his mind without his volition, from outside himself ... [T]here is a clearly a disturbance in the self-image, and especially in the boundary between what is self and what is not self; thoughts which have in fact arisen inside himself are considered to have been inserted into his thinking from outside: 'A 29 year old housewife said, "I look out of the window and I think the garden looks nice and the grass looks cool, but the thoughts of Eamonn Andrews come into my mind. There are no other thoughts there,

only his ... He treats my mind like a screen and flashes his thoughts onto it like you flash a picture". (Sims 1988: 122)

In fact, the view that there is an error about the boundaries of the mind has been contested (Stephens and Graham 1994). However, what does seem to be key is that subjects of thought insertion have a delusion about agency: somehow they do not believe that they are the active thinkers of thoughts that they have.

Thought insertion presents a phenomenologically-minded approach to psychopathology with a particularly clear instance of a general problem discussed in Chapter 3. How can we make sense of psychopathological states and experiences that defy everyday interpretation or recontextualisation? The delusional belief that thoughts are entering a subject's mind from an outside source is not merely false but altogether bizarre. Why do sufferers non-collusively report experiences of this extraordinary form? What exactly do they believe about the boundaries of their inner space or, perhaps better, of agency?

Shedding some light on the phenomenon of thought insertions could take two (non-exclusive) forms. On the one hand, its occurrence might be explained by discovering more about its aetiology, its causal antecedents and the physiological mechanisms involved. On the other, light might be shed on the *content* of the delusion, on what sufferers actually believe and the rational structure (to the extent that there is one) of that belief. Putting this point in this way stresses the differences between what might be called—following in the tradition of psychopathology—the distinction between reasons and causes.

A cognitivist approach promises to shed light in both of these ways. As the cognitive neurologist Chris Frith says:

> My approach will be to develop as complete as possible an explanation at the psychological level. In parallel with this there should eventually be a complete explanation at the physiological level. Both explanations should be continuously modified so that mapping from one to another is made easier ... Given this approach to the relationship between mind and brain, there are two clear components in any attempt to specify the neuropsychology of schizophrenia. First, a description of schizophrenic abnormalities at a psychological level, and, second, a specification of how this description maps onto abnormalities at a physiological level. (Frith 1992: 27–9)

In line with this general strategy, cognitivist accounts of the mind attempt to describe and (partially) explain psychopathology by articulating mental functions in information processing terms and describing their systematic relations. As I will describe below, a cognitivist account of thought insertion is then made possible by describing a breakdown of a self-monitoring mechanism of mental representations which are then experienced as alien.

Cognitivism thus looks to provide a plausible account of thought insertion because it relies on what can be characterised as an 'alienated' conception of thoughts as internal mental representations. However, as I have argued in the previous section, there is something wrong with the very idea of mental states as part of inner space. At the very least, it calls for a further account of how cognitivist accounts of meaning are supposed to function. In this section, I will argue that the very ease with which cognitivism characterises the abnormal phenomenon of thought insertion suggests there is something wrong with its account of normality. Whilst deploying a literally spatial conception of inner space appears to shed light on what might metaphorically be described as a disorder of inner space that move is, in fact, disastrous.

The cognitivist framework provides what seems at first to be an attractive account of thought insertion, as well as other passivity phenomena such as 'made actions' in which subjects experience actions as somehow not their own. (In 'Free will in the light of neuropsychiatry' the psychiatrist Sean Spence usefully summarises a number of brief case vignettes (Spence 1996).) What is most paradoxical about thought insertion, for example, is the very idea of the subject of a thought, the person capable of expressing it, coming 'adrift' from it and finding it alien. Frith's general idea in *The Cognitive Neuropsychology of Schizophrenia* is to explain the delusion of thought insertion as an understandable belief in response to an abnormal experience (see the discussion of Maher in Chapter 3). What seems to be a paradoxical disorder of inner space is explained through a particular scientific model of inner states.

Frith adds to the cognitivist picture of the mind so far discussed a further information processing idea: the idea of monitoring and labelling one's thoughts. Drawing on the idea of a mechanism of 'corollary discharge' or 're-afference copy' more usually described in the case of eye movements to distinguish the experience of moving one's eyes from the case of the world moving, Frith suggests that similar mechanisms apply in general to mental states (Frith 1992: 81). Such monitoring is not only involved in distinguishing actions from what is done to a subject. It also plays a role in identifying thoughts:

> I believe that it is not only monitoring of action that is impaired in schizophrenia. In addition, it is the monitoring of the intentions to act. I am essentially describing two steps in a central monitoring system. First, the relation between actions and external events are monitored ... Second, intentions are monitored in order to distinguish between actions caused by our own goals and plans (willed actions) and actions that are in response to external events (stimulus-driven actions). Such monitoring is essential if we are to have awareness of the causes of our actions ... A failure to monitor intentions to act would result in delusions of control and other passivity experiences. Thinking, like all our actions, is normally accompanied by a sense of effort and deliberate choice as we move from one thought to the next. If we found ourselves thinking without any awareness of the sense of effort that reflects central monitoring we might well experience these thoughts as alien and, thus, being inserted into our minds.

Similarly actions would appear to be determined by external forces if there was no awareness of the intention to act. (Frith 1992: 81–2)

The main attraction of this picture is this. If mental states are described as free-standing states then it seems to be a contingent matter how their ownership is established. Thus, it seems to be quite comprehensible that one might have a state whose ownership is not satisfactorily settled by an inner monitoring mechanism and is thus experienced as imposed from without. (Frith does not attempt a full answer as to why it is often ascribed to particular others.) However, the very ease with which thought insertion can be interpreted on this general picture suggests that the picture itself is wrong.

As a preliminary, note first the kind of account sketched out in the quotation above. It is pitched at a psychological level and its initial plausibility (its face validity) flows from that. The states that are monitored include *intentions*: everyday folk psychological states. *Monitoring* is the sort of activity in which one can consciously engage. One might attempt to monitor the regularity of one's breathing or heart rate, or the number of times one's thoughts turn unbidden to Buffy the Vampire Slayer.

It is thus relevant to examine how phenomenologically plausible this sort of account is. Frith says that 'thinking, like all our actions, is normally accompanied by a sense of effort and deliberate choice as we move from one thought to the next'. This is not an entirely natural description of thought, however. Whilst there may sometimes be a *sense of effort* involved in thinking through an issue or keeping one's thoughts focused on a tedious problem, much thought has no such quality. This is not to say that thought is not a matter of *deliberate choice*. One can choose to think through an issue, for example, although one's thoughts can also turn 'unbidden' in a new direction. (What is particularly interesting about Spence's 1996 paper is the suggestion of some phenomenological continuity between everyday spontaneous thought and thought insertion.) Nevertheless, what does *not* follow is that deliberate choice in one's mental processes corresponds to a sense of effort.

In addition to criticism of the plausibility of the details of the phenomenological account, I want to raise two structural difficulties. The first concerns how, once an alienated conception of mental states is in play, it is reined in in normal cases. The second concerns its inability to find paradoxical a family of claims that do seem to be paradoxes. In both cases, the problem stems from the alienated conception of thoughts as inner states. Thus, the general difficulty with cognitivism described in the previous section gives rise to a related specific difficulty in the case of thought insertion.

Frith's account of made actions, actions experienced as somehow not a subject's own, is this. A subject acts, but does not experience her intention to act and, thus, experiences the act as alien and attributes it to an outside source. An experience of thought insertion results from the subject not experiencing a thought as her own. The latter case is expressed in the quotation above: 'If we found ourselves thinking without any awareness of the sense of effort that reflects central monitoring we might well experience these thoughts as alien and, thus, being inserted into our minds'. This suggests that in non-pathological cases it is precisely having an experience of a sense of effort that enables a subject to identify a thought as her own.

Presumably, the sense of effort is also to be explained in cognitivist terms: as an inner state encoding a sense of effort as its content. This then raises the further question: if the difference between an experience of thought insertion and a non-pathological case turns on the having of a sense of effort, how is the sense of effort identified as the subject's own? The problem is structural. It stems from the fact that inner states are not essentially owned (or, perhaps, experienced as essentially owned) and, thus, have to be possessed via a further state or experience that labels them as owned by the subject. However, given Frith's general explanatory framework, the question of ownership (or the experience of ownership) will return to the sense of effort that is supposed to label the original thought. How is the sense of effort owned? Is there a further sense of effort attached to having whatever mental representation encodes the first sense of effort attached to having the original thought? If so, a vicious regress beckons.

Whilst cognitivism is a thoroughly modern form of materialism, the objection I have just sketched out is of the same form as the Oxford philosopher Gilbert Ryle's (1900–1976) objection to the broadly Cartesian 'Myth of Volitions' in his influential book *The Concept of Mind* (Ryle 1949). Within the kind of account he attacks, volitions are deployed to explain the difference between actions and mere movements. According to the myth, bodily actions are those bodily movements that originate from volitions, which are themselves mental efficient causes. Given that the kind of purposive descriptions which apply to bodily actions can also apply to mental operations, this raises the question of the status of volitions. Are they voluntary or involuntary acts of mind? (ibid: 65). If volitions are involuntary then they do not explain how the acts that result from them are voluntary. If they are voluntary then, given the explanatory framework in place, that will require a vicious regress of further volitions. The inner states postulated by cognitivism are not immaterial, as volitions were supposed to be, but they suffer some of the same structural defects nevertheless.

The second structural difficulty I wish to flag is broader. It concerns the Cambridge philosopher G. E. Moore's (1873–1958) famous paradox: 'It is raining, but I do not believe it'. Note that it would *not* be paradoxical to say 'it is raining but you do not believe it'; or 'it was raining but I did not believe it'.

Nevertheless, the first statement is, in Moore's phrase, 'absurd'. Now there is disagreement about the analysis of the statement and thus just why exactly it is paradoxical. (Wittgenstein discusses it at some length in his *Remarks on the Philosophy of Psychology* (Wittgenstein 1980)). But most accounts are based on the idea that the first person present tense 'I believe that p' functions very like 'p' and thus that the paradox is of the form 'p and not p'. Whatever the analysis, however, it does seem to be a feature of our concept of belief that Moore's statement is a paradox. Thus, a broadly psychological account of belief that could not account for the paradoxical quality of this statement would be *prima facie* implausible. That, however, is a problem for cognitivism. The problem is that if inner states are self-ascribed through a monitoring process, then it seems merely contingent that the state of affairs reported in Moore's statement is not more widely reported. It seems that it should, at the very least, be thinkable.

The self-report expressed in Moore's paradox is close cousin of the reports which characterise thought insertion. This suggests that there is the following pay-off. A cognitivist account of monitoring inner states promises to explain the pathological case, but only at the cost of making the everyday paradoxical nature of Moore's statement mysterious instead. An alienated account of a subject's relation to her thoughts would indeed make thought insertion more comprehensible but only at the cost of making our normal connection to our mental states the more baffling.

As I have argued above, there are two related problems for cognitivist accounts of the mind. Both turn on the construal of mental states as inner states that encode information or contents in accord with a computational, information processing account of the mind. The first concerns the severing of the subject from the world. The second concerns the severing of the subject from her own thoughts. In both cases, it may be possible to describe further mechanisms to reattach subject and world or subject and thought, but it is an open question whether this strategy will address the real source of problem, which is the cognitivist framework and its appeal to a literal construal of the mind as inner space.

If not cognitivism, what account can be given of meaning? The next section of this chapter will develop an answer to that question by examining a version of discursive psychology based on a social constructionist account of meaning. I will argue that approach is also deeply flawed, but that it helps point towards a proper conception of meaning, which will be developed in the third section.

It is worth flagging here, however, some unfinished business. What account can be given of the functional dependence diagrams that are popularised by cognitivist accounts of mind? If the idea that meanings are carried by inner states is rejected, can an account be given of such depictions of relations between mental modules? I will sketch a brief answer to that question at the end of the chapter.

## 2. The discursive turn, social constructionism and dementia

In addition to, and in competition with, cognitivist accounts of meaning within psychiatry there is a second influential approach to meaning within mental health care: discursive psychology. This second section will outline the motivations for discursive psychology and its connections to social constructionism. I will then explain how an interpretation of Wittgenstein is supposed to underpin constructionism but, in fact, does not do so. The third section of the chapter will then describe an alternative, Wittgenstein-inspired approach, which aims to naturalise meaning without reducing it to purely causal or law-like terms.

A discursive approach to the mind has a number of attractions. Centrally, it places meaning in the public world. This helps sidestep a worry that might otherwise arise about the privacy of meaning and a version of the problem of other minds. The discursive view thus makes a phenomenon, which we generally take for granted outside, perhaps, clinical circumstances, more explicable. In general, we can know or have 'access' to other people's meanings. We do generally know what other people mean. If meaning, by contrast with a discursive approach, is thought of as a matter of an internal state of mind then substantial further work has to be done to show how this could be shared. The discursive approach, instead, starts with a picture of meaning as essentially sharable and, thus, no such subsequent explanatory work has to be done.

A discursive view also helps place meaning in nature. This is a point to which I shall return, but preliminarily, it helps to show that meaning is a perfectly natural aspect of the world that fits into an everyday conception of reality. However—and this will become an important point—it does not do this by relating it to a more basic natural scientific world view. At its best, it is a form of naturalism without being a form of reductionist naturalism. I will argue, however, that, in its own way, a social constructionist view of discursive psychology is a form of reductionist naturalism, although it does not aim to reduce meaning to states within the head.

In mental health care, especially dementia, a discursive view encourages a person-centred interpretational approach exemplified in the work of the psychologists Steven Sabat and Tom Kitwood, rather than the 'defectological' view in which 'the afflicted person is defined principally in terms of his or her catalogued dysfunctions' (Sabat 2001: 10).

In the case of dementia, a discursive approach may have a fourth further attraction. This depends on a connection between the discursive turn and constructionism that will be outlined in the next two sub-sections. By 'constructionism' I mean the view that meanings are constituted by ongoing linguistic moves, rather than the ongoing linguistic moves being governed by antecedent meanings. If the discursive approach is also constructionist then the following possibility arises. The assumption that meanings are constructed in ongoing conversations, need not imply that all parties in the conversation take on equal conversational work in their construction. Thus, it might seem that there can be compensation where one party is no longer equally able to take part through, for example, the onset of dementia. The philosopher Jennifer Radden and psychotherapist Joan Fordyce articulate just this view. They say:

> The model of collective identity sustenance requires others to do more and to do it differently ... Increasingly, others must remember, reinforce, and reinscribe the identity of the person with dementia ... The construction and sustaining of the person's characterization identity have been, until the deficits of dementia make themselves known, collective efforts conducted largely tacitly. Increasingly, as these deficits erode aspects of the person's memory and self-awareness, the task will come to include the provision of explicit identity recognition ... Until now, also, to the extent that others were called on to sustain the identities of those around them, this task will have been largely mutual ... Now, however, the task of holding and preserving identity of the person suffering dementia will come to be placed squarely on the shoulders of others. (Radden and Fordyce 2006: 80–1)

Now there is an everyday sense in which this seems perfectly plausible. It is a matter of phenomenological fact that one can work to make sense of utterances, which are not initially clear. On a constructionist view, however, this flows from a deep feature of meaning—the fact that it is of its very nature to be invented piecemeal. The work is not one of detection of meaning, but co-creation. Whilst I do not want to cast doubt on the phenomenological fact just mentioned, I do intend to dispute this explanation of it.

Nevertheless, if it is to be a genuine alternative to the cognitivist orthodoxy, the discursive approach has to make a stronger claim than that meanings are caused by social factors and constructionism is one way to discharge that obligation. So, if not constructionism, then what? In the third part of this chapter I will return to this question and briefly outline the resources for a non-constructionist version of discursive psychology.

## The discursive turn and its contrast with cognitivism

In this subsection I shall outline the discursive approach to psychology or psychiatry, contrasting it with cognitivism, explain the importance of the distinction between constitutive and causal accounts of the role of social factors, and describe the connection between the discursive turn and social constructionism.

Discursive psychology is the name of a family of approaches taken by different authors, who share the central assumption that psychological phenomena can be investigated through the analysis of 'discourse'. The focus on discourse, as opposed to language, marks the fact that 'discourse is to be treated as a social practice which can be studied as a real-world phenomenon rather than a theoretical abstraction' (Edwards and Potter 1992: 15). Thus, the focus is on actual utterances, rather than the structure of rules or grammar that make up a language. Discursive psychology is based on the central idea that 'some central psychological phenomena are related in participants' discourse' (Edwards and Potter 1992: 1–2). However, as I shall describe, this is not supposed to be merely a heuristic device, but a radical theoretical perspective.

Edwards and Potter explicitly contrast their own approach in *Discursive Psychology* with a 'cognitivist' approach:

> A contrast is drawn between cognitivist approaches to language, where texts, sentences and descriptions are taken as ... realizations of underlying cognitive representations of ... [the] world; and the discursive approach where versions of events, things, people and so on, are studied and theorized primarily in terms of how those versions are constructed in an occasioned manner to accomplish social actions. (Edwards and Potter 1992: 8)

Whilst cognitivism takes utterances to be expressions of and thus depend on mental states, construed as underlying representations, a discursive approach inverts the priority and, instead, regards psychological phenomena as dependent on, and explicable in terms of, the social phenomena of language use, action and so on.

As I explained earlier in this chapter, a key element of cognitivism is that for information (or 'content' as it also known) to be processed there have to be bearers of that information (or content). Thus, the mind or brain is populated with states or 'representations' (as in the quotation from Edwards and Potter above) that carry meaning or encode content. A computational approach to the mind presupposes a medium of computation: a system of inner states or representations. Thus, states of mind are constituted, according to this view, by internal information-bearing states of the brain or nervous system. In other words, they are constituted by factors within the skull. Utterances and other 'outer' behaviour are merely evidence for the inner states that causes them. A discursive approach, by contrast, inverts the priority of mind and linguistic behaviour presupposed by cognitivism. Psychological phenomena are constituted, in some way yet to be determined, by linguistic phenomena, by utterances or conversations.

One advantage of the discursive approach from a philosophical perspective is that it undercuts a worry about the privacy of meanings and mental states that might otherwise exist and which is encouraged by a cognitivist approach. If mental states are construed as internal states of a person, then a number of problems arise. First, there is the problem of other minds: how do we know what mental states others are in if all we have to base our judgements on are outward appearances? Secondly, how do we know what others mean if meanings are, again, internal matters? Thirdly, if our own mental states are also internal states, how can they reveal the outer world? Why are we not trapped within a 'veil of perceptions'?

The discursive turn, by contrast, attempts to sidestep the problem of connecting inner states to the world—and thus accounting for intentionality—by placing meaning firmly in the public realm. Broadly, if meaning is constituted in public interactions then the challenge to bridge a gap between the inner and the outer, the private and the public, falls away. The materials on which an account of meaning is to be based are always already outer and public. (There may be a corresponding problem, however, of explaining how one knows one's own state of mind. Connecting mind to the outer world threatens to sever its connection to the subject or person.)

The putative advantages of discursive psychology are mentioned by Harré and Gillett in *The Discursive Mind*:

> Obviously the things that fix the meanings of words cannot be hidden inside the respective heads of different people or else we would each be uncertain all the time what anybody else was talking about. Thus it is hard to say what I could mean by claiming that my thoughts are true, and my utterances meaningful, if I am trapped within them and at their mercy (and they are hidden inside me). The problem runs very deep because others cannot get outside their veils of perception either. This entails that none of us knows what the world is really like, nor what others think, nor whether anything we think is actually true, nor what anyone else means by the words they use, nor indeed what I mean by the words I use. Clearly, we have to find some way to make sense of the fact that we *can* aim to think true thoughts and express them in a common system of signs. This is an even more pressing need when we consider the fact that thoughts are communicable. (Harré and Gillett 1994: 43)

A discursive approach thus seems to have a fundamental advantage concerning the metaphysics and epistemology of mind, but if it really has these advantages it must be genuinely distinct from cognitivism. It must amount to a *constitutive*, rather than a merely causal claim about the connection of mind and discourse. Even a cognitivist can accept, for example, that mental states or meanings are caused by social factors. He or she can take a wider view of the influences on psychological phenomena than one which restricts itself to what happens within the skull, but that is consistent with also holding, as cognitivists typically do, that such effects are mediated by what happens within the skull.

To be genuinely distinct, the discursive approach must involve a claim that psychological phenomena are not merely caused by social factors, but also constituted by them, rather than constituted by factors within the skull. This is suggested by Harré and Gillett:

> In this sense, the psychological is not reducible to or replaceable by explanations in terms of physiology, physics, or any other point of view that does not reveal the structure of meanings existing in the lives of the human group to which the subject of an investigation belongs. (Harré and Gillett 1994: 20)

By claiming that that the psychological is irreducible, they suggest a stronger claim than the mere causal role of social factors. They summarize their view thus:

1. Many psychological phenomena are to be interpreted as properties or features of discourse, and that discourse might be public or private. As public, it is behaviour; as private, it is thought.
2. Individual and private uses of symbolic systems, which in this view constitute thinking, are derived from interpersonal discursive processes that are the main feature of the human environment.
3. The production of psychological phenomena, such as emotions, decisions, attitudes, personality displays, and so on, in discourse depends upon the skill of the actors, their relative moral standing in the community, and the story lines that unfold. (Harré and Gillett 1994: 27)

Whilst this characterization is not completely clear, it contains a good indication of a constitutive view. Psychological factors are construed as aspects of discourse itself. Thinking comprises private discourse—'individual and private uses of symbol systems'—but this is, in turn, derived from interpersonal processes. Psychological phenomena are not merely produced *by* discourse—as a cognitivist might agree when, for example, anger, construed as an inner state, is caused by harsh words—but produced *in* the discourse. The idea of 'private uses' or the claim that 'discourse ... as private ... is thought' is not completely straightforward, but, nevertheless, the approach summarized looks to be genuinely distinct from a form of cognitivism, whether or not it is ultimately coherent.

So far I have highlighted the central role that public utterance plays in discursive psychology and contrasted it with cognitivism. I have stressed the claim that it has to be a constitutive rather than a causal account of the mind if it is to be genuinely distinct from cognitivism. This leaves, however, the question of how that constitutive claim is unpacked. What exactly is the constitutive claim? How does discourse constitute psychological phenomena?

The most common answer to this question adopted by the discursive turn is a form of social constructionism. If psychological phenomena, including mental states and meanings, are constructed by utterances then this both explains the constitutive connection, and also underpins a clear distinction between discursive psychology and cognitivism. (On the latter view, by contrast, utterances are merely evidence of pre-existing underlying states, which do not depend constitutively on them.) The constructionist view of discursive psychology is expressed in the following passages:

> In this view, our delineation of the subject matter of psychology has to take account of discourses, significations, subjectivities, and positionings, for it is in these that psychological phenomena *actually* exist. For example, an attitude should not be seen as a semi-permanent mental entity, causing people to say and do certain things, rather, it *comes into existence* in displays expressive of decisions and judgments and in the performance of actions. (Harré and Gillett 1994: 22 italics added)

> In keeping with the discursive approach to psychology, this study is based on the principle that meanings are jointly constituted by participants in a conversation.
>
> From the discursive point of view, psychological phenomena are not inner or hidden properties or processes of mind which discourse merely expresses. The discursive expression is … the psychological phenomenon itself …
>
> Personhood can be an interpersonal discursive construction, a property of conversations …
>
> "The mind" is no more than, but no less than, a privatised part of the "general conversation". Meanings are jointly constructed by competent actors in the course of projects that are realised within systems of public norms. (Sabat and Harré 1994: 144–6)

> [R]ather than seeing such discursive constructions as expressions of speakers' underlying cognitive states, they are examined in the context of their occurrence as situated and occasioned constructions whose precise nature makes sense, to participants and analysts alike, in terms of the social actions those descriptions accomplish. (Edwards and Potter 1992: 2)

The broad thrust of these accounts of the discursive approach is that it is based on the constitution of psychological phenomena in utterances and other social actions, and these construct the phenomena in question. The constitutive claim that helps distinguish a discursive approach from cognitivism is underpinned by a constructionist claim. If psychological phenomena are constructed in, for example, ongoing conversations, then they cannot be constituted by states within the skull.

There is a further characterisation of constructionist forms of discursive psychology that will be useful later. It is best described through a contrast, again, with cognitivism. A cognitivist approach aims to fit meaning and mental states within a broadly natural scientific account of the world in general, and psychiatry and mental health in particular. It is thus a form of naturalism in its reductionist form: the same form as descriptivist accounts of illness took in Chapter 1. The problematic and puzzling phenomena of meaning are to be shown to be natural and thus not, in fact, puzzling by relating them to paradigmatically natural phenomena. The puzzling phenomena are explained in more basic terms and thus reduced to them. Of course, it is a matter of decision what the paradigmatically natural phenomena are. Jerry Fodor, for example, selects the catalogue that *physicists* have been compiling 'of the ultimate and irreducible properties of things' (Fodor 1987: 97). But, the aim of making sense of puzzling phenomena, of making them natural, takes the form of an explanation in more basic terms.

Given that it resists reduction of psychological phenomena to what lies within the skull, discursive psychology seems to stand opposed to that picture. Indeed, two social psychologists Dian-Marie Hosking and Ian Morley make this point explicitly:

> 'Social constructionism' (as we see it) refers to a loose concatenation of theoretical frameworks that emphasise *both* the constructive powers of human minds and their origins in conversations, conventions, and cultural traditions … Such frameworks have developed from long-standing philosophical traditions, and they provide a background to at least two contemporary debates: one that contrasts psychology as a natural science with psychology as a moral science, and one that contrasts individual psychology with collective psychology. Often, but not always, those who see psychology as a natural science want to reduce social psychology to individual psychology. Often, but not always, those who see psychology as a moral science see psychology as concerned with reasons rather than causes and with forms of self-expression that are constituted in conversations, unique to certain times and places. (Hosking and Morley 2004: 318–9)

Hosking and Morley thus suggest that social constructionism—and by implication a constructionist form of discursive psychology—stands opposed to the reductionist naturalism that grounds cognitivism. Whereas cognitivism aims to fit mind and meaning into a natural scientific account, social constructionism aims to deny that and, possibly, to see psychology as a moral science rather than a natural science. Whilst I agree that this is an important aspect of a broadly discursive approach, I shall argue shortly that constructionism in fact shares some aspect of the reductionist naturalist approach and that discursive psychology is better purged of that reductionist aspiration.

If the discursive turn is underpinned by a form of social constructionism then, whatever its methodological fruitfulness in empirical investigation, it is a radical and counter-intuitive account of the mind. This prompts the question: is it tenable? One key influence on social constructionist accounts of meaning has been a family of interpretations of Wittgenstein to which I shall now turn to assess this question.

## Wittgenstein and constructionism about meaning

In this subsection I shall briefly summarize a familiar argument for a social constructionist view of meaning drawn from Wittgenstein (for a longer treatment see Thornton 1998). This is the second appearance that Wittgenstein's discussion makes in this book (see also Chapters 2 and 6). Here, I shall examine its consequences for constructionist accounts of meaning.

Wittgenstein's discussion of rules, which lies at the heart of his *Philosophical Investigations*, has been taken by a number of authors to support a form of social constructionism about meaning. Rules and meanings are connected because meanings are normative. To understand the meaning of a word is to understand how to use it correctly. It is to understand the rule that prescribes its correct use. So an account of understanding rules in general will shed light on understanding meanings. The analysis will also have consequences for mental content—the 'meaning' of mental states—because that is also normative.

The problem that Wittgenstein introduces at the start of the discussion of rules follows from two features of understanding:

> But we *understand* the meaning of a word when we hear or say it; we grasp it in a flash, and what we grasp in this way is surely something different from the 'use' which is extended in time! (Wittgenstein 1953: §138)

> [I]sn't the meaning of the word also determined by this use? And can these ways of determining meaning conflict? Can what we grasp *in a flash* accord with a use, fit or fail to fit it? And how can what is present to us in an instant, what comes before our mind in an instant, fit a *use*? (Wittgenstein 1953: §139)

Understanding a rule (such as the circumstances for the correct application of a word or for the equally open-ended continuation of a mathematical series) can be both manifested over time, but also expressed at a particular time, when one grasps how to go on, perhaps exclaiming 'Now I've got it!' If understanding has these two aspects, what is it that connects them?

Later in the *Investigations*, Wittgenstein describes a related puzzle concerning the intentionality of mental content more generally:

> A wish seems already to know what will or would satisfy it; a proposition, a thought, what makes it true—even when that thing is not there at all! Whence this *determining* of what is not yet there? This despotic demand? (Wittgenstein 1953: §437).

Again the question is what connects a state at one time with the worldly feature it is about (and sometimes even a feature that does not exist)?

The most promising approach to the question seems to be to sketch a mental mechanism that connects an initial experience or state of grasping a rule with its subsequent correct application. Wittgenstein, however, considers and rejects a number of plausible mechanisms. None can support the normative connection between understanding a rule or the meaning of a word and its correct application. (Similarly, no mechanism can connect an intentional mental state and what it is about.)

Saul Kripke, in an influential account of these sections, highlights Wittgenstein's criticism of theories that implicitly rely on an act of interpretation. It is tempting to think that understanding consists in something coming before the mind's eye, something like a symbol or picture. If, however, understanding were to consist in entertaining an inner symbol then it would do so only under a particular interpretation of that symbol. If understanding is a form of interpretation, the correct interpretation of the symbol would also have to be codified in a further inner symbol that would, in turn, require further interpretation. Thus, a vicious regress begins. It is vicious because the first symbol only has any meaning under an interpretation specified by the completed infinite series of further interpretations.

Kripke reinforces this argument by postulating a sceptic who challenges us to justify our normal pre-philosophical claim to know which arithmetical rules we have followed in the past, specifically using, as an example, addition. He postulates a sceptical alternative: a deviant version of addition that differs only in cases not so far considered. The challenge is to show that we have always added in the past rather than used the deviant or 'bent' function. The problem is that any previous statement we may have made of the rule, or any finite behavioural evidence for it, or any mental images that might depict it, can be interpreted in more than one way: in accord with both addition and the deviant rule (which differs only in cases so far not considered). Thus, it seems that we cannot defeat a sceptical challenge to our claim to understand what rule we have followed in the past, but nothing is different about the present case. Kripke concludes that this undermines the very idea of determinate meanings. He is a kind of sceptic about meaning:

> There can be no such thing as meaning anything by any word. Each new application we make is a leap in the dark; any present intention could be interpreted so as to accord with anything we may choose to do. So there can be neither accord, nor conflict. This is what Wittgenstein said in §202 [sic]. (Kripke 1982: 55)

In its place he deploys a form of social constructionism:

> It is essential to our concept of a rule that we maintain some such conditional as 'If Jones means addition by "+", then if he is asked for "68 + 57", he will reply "125"'… [T]he conditional as stated makes it appear that some mental state obtains in Jones that guarantees his performance of particular additions such as '68 + 57'—just what the sceptical argument denies. Wittgenstein's picture of the true situation concentrates on the contrapositive, and on justification conditions. If Jones does *not* come out with '125' when asked about '68 + 57', we cannot assert that he means addition by '+'. (Kripke 1982: 94–5)

Kripke's suggestion is that whilst rules cannot prescribe their correct applications, there can be the appearance of rule-governed behaviour, and thus of meaning, providing that there is a community. The community provides a negative standard by which ongoing practice can be judged. As long as he or she is not criticized by the community a subject can be considered to be following a rule.

Thus, something like correctness is constituted by the ongoing judgements of the community.

Kripke is not the only philosopher to offer an explicitly constructionist view of meaning. Although he criticizes Kripke's sceptical argument, Crispin Wright also deploys a form of constructionism. According to Wright:

> One of the most basic philosophical puzzles about intentional states is that they seem to straddle two conflicting paradigms: on the one hand they are avowable, so to that extent conform to the paradigm of sensation and other 'observable' phenomena of consciousness; on the other they answer constitutively to the ways in which the subject manifests them, and to that extent conform to the paradigm of psychological characteristics which, like irritability or modesty, are properly conceived as dispositional ... It seems that neither an epistemology of observation—of pure introspection—nor one of inference can be harmonised with all aspects of the intentional. (Wright 1991: 142)

Intention is only one example of a general phenomenon which also includes understanding, remembering and deciding. In each case, a subject has a special non-inferential authority in ascribing these to herself, which is, nevertheless, defeasible in the light of subsequent performance. Wittgenstein's attack on explanations of such states shows that they cannot be modelled on a Cartesian picture of observation of inner experiences (because such inner states cannot prescribe what should satisfy them). But if understanding, intending and the like are to be modelled on abilities instead, as Wittgenstein seems to suggest, how can the subject have special authority in ascribing these to herself in the light of the attack on substantial explanation?

Constructivism appears to provide a solution to this problem. The basic idea is to deny that there is any inner epistemology and to devise a constructivist account of intention instead:

> The authority which our self-ascriptions of meaning, intention, and decision assume is not based on any kind of cognitive advantage, expertise or achievement. Rather it is, as it were, a *concession*, unofficially granted to anyone whom one takes seriously as a rational subject. It is, so to speak, such a subject's right to declare what he intends, what he intended, and what satisfies his intentions; and his possession of this right consists in the conferral upon such declarations, other things being equal, of a *constitutive* rather than descriptive role. (Wright 1987: 400)

All other things being equal, a speaker's sincere judgements constitute the content of the intention, understanding or decision. They determine, rather than reflect, the content of the state concerned. The meaning of a word or the content of an intention is constituted by the ongoing judgements a speaker makes. Elsewhere, Wright talks of meaning as being 'plastic in response to speakers' ongoing performance' (Wright 1986: 289).

Although constructionist interpretations of Wittgenstein have been influential, there is mounting reason to doubt that they are a satisfactory interpretation. The central philosophical objection to constructionism about meaning is that it fails in its main aim. It attempts to explain a problematic concept—in this case meaning or content including, centrally, its normativity—in simpler terms. In this aim, it is a form of reductionist naturalism like cognitivist accounts of meaning, or descriptivist accounts of illness discussed in Chapter 1. Having found the notion of understanding a rule (that prescribes correct use) or forming an intention (that prescribes what should satisfy it) puzzling, it attempts to rebuild that notion from more basic ideas. Kripke aims to capture an ersatz notion of the normativity of rules using the idea of (absence of) communal dissent. We are justified in ascribing accord with a rule to a subject providing that they have not disagreed with the community. Wright aims to capture the normativity of mental content such as the content of intentions using a subject's ongoing avowals or judgements.

There are two main problems with the approach. First, neither Kripke nor Wright succeeds in re-capturing the pre-philosophical notion that such judgements answer to something, and that has radical and implausible consequences. To take just one key problem, without the notion that there is something that it would be correct to assert in a circumstance, we lose the right to think of states or affairs or facts that are independent of judgement. If so, such constructionism leads to a crude idealism.

Secondly, the approach is inconsistent in that both Kripke and Wright appeal to notions of meaning or content in their attempt to explain it. Kripke appeals to dissent, Wright to individual judgment. But both of these notions require prior grasp of norms: the norms governing the meaning of 'no', perhaps, and governing the content of individual judgments that are supposed to 'unpack' or construct the content of intentions, respectively.

It is also important to keep in mind how constructionism falsifies everyday phenomenology. As McDowell asserts:

> But suppose I form the intention to type a period. If that is my intention, it is settled that only my typing a period will count as executing it. Of course I am capable of forming that intention only because I am party to the practices that are constitutive of the relevant concepts. But if that is indeed the intention that—thus empowered—I form, nothing more than the intention itself is needed to determine what counts as conformity to it. Certainly it needs no help from my subsequent judgements. (Suppose I forgot what a period is.) So there is something for my intention to type a period, conceived as determining what counts as conformity to it autonomously and independently of my judgements on the matter, to be: namely, precisely, my intention to type a period … This is common sense, not platonism. (McDowell 1998b: 315)

This criticism of a constructivist account turns, however, on the absence of an alternative. If Kripke's reading of Wittgenstein were correct then a merely ersatz version of meaning might be the best that were possible. Thus, the criticism that constructionism does not succeed in capturing our pre-philosophical notions of meaning only has bite if there is an alternative interpretation of Wittgenstein's negative view.

In fact there is. As McDowell convincingly argues, Wittgenstein's critical arguments are directed not against meaning itself, but against a particular philosophical explanation of it. Crucially, such explanations form what we might call the Cartesian 'master thesis':

> We get a more radical divergence from Kripke, however, if we suppose that the thrust of Wittgenstein's reflections is to cast doubt on the master thesis: the thesis that whatever a person has in her mind, it is only by virtue of being interpreted in one of various possible ways that it can impose a sorting of extra-mental items into those that accord with it and those that do not.
>
> It is really an extraordinary idea that the contents of minds are things that, considered in themselves, just "stand there". We can bring out how extraordinary it is by noting that we need an application for the concept of accord, and so run the risk of trouble from the regress of interpretations if we accept the master thesis, not just in connection with grasp of meaning, but in connection with intentionality in general. An intention, just as such, is something with which only acting in a specific way would accord. An expectation, just as such, is something with which only certain future states of affairs would accord. Quite generally, a thought, just as such, is something with which only certain states of affairs would accord. (McDowell 1998b: 270)

Thus, the assumption that understanding is a form of interpretation is an instance of the master thesis that the mind is populated with items which merely can be interpreted as relating to the world. Rejecting that thesis, a thesis also held by cognitivist approaches to the mind, undermines the attraction of a social constructionist approach to meaning and mental states. It is the assumption that the only things that can come before the mind are free-standing and thus need to be interpreted to be about anything that makes the only perceived alternative—that meaning is made up, piecemeal, in discursive practice—attractive. Rejecting that assumption—a hidden agreement between cognitivism and constructionism—leaves space for the everyday idea that in speaking one expresses and answers to the meaning of words and, equally, that one can put one's antecedent thoughts into words. There is thus no need for the reconstructive philosophy explicit in social constructionist forms of discursive psychology.

This section has outlined the attractions of social constructionism in discursive psychology. It is a view that suggests that minds and meanings are essentially public phenomena and thus undercuts potential concerns that other people's minds are private and inaccessible. It is often thought to be supported by the later Wittgenstein's discussion of rule following. I have argued, however, that the view is untenable. Furthermore, properly understood, arguments from Wittgenstein undermine, rather than support constructionism. This raises the question: what positive account of mental content and linguistic meaning does Wittgenstein suggest for mental health care?

## 3. A Wittgensteinian account of meaning

This section will develop the account of Wittgenstein so far given to sketch a positive view of both linguistic meaning and mental content. I will begin by articulating a brief positive account of both meaning and mental content drawn from the later Wittgenstein. The middle two subsections will critically examine the different use that Derek Bolton and Jonathan Hill make of Wittgenstein. Finally, I will return to consider the view of discursive psychology that is best supported by philosophical considerations.

I have argued in the first two sections of this chapter that cognitivism (or representationalism) and constructivism share a key assumption. They assume that the meaning of linguistic signs should be explained as resulting either from prior mental acts or from social processes, which can also be characterised independently of the content that they are supposed to explain. As Wittgenstein argues, however, once understanding is equated with a free-standing mental state or process, nothing can reconnect that state to future acts. Once a social process is described in terms that are not explicitly normative, it cannot be used to explain meaning which is essentially normative.

Having summarised the unsuccessful strategy for explaining the normative connections a rule has with its correct applications, Wittgenstein comments:

> What this shews is that there is a way of grasping a rule which is *not* an *interpretation*, but which is exhibited in what we call 'obeying the rule' and 'going against it' in actual cases. (Wittgenstein 1953: §201)

> And hence also 'obeying a rule' is a practice. And to *think* one is obeying a rule is not to obey a rule. (Wittgenstein 1953: §202)

At first sight invoking practice may seem neither radical nor helpful. The whole of the practice of correctly using a word can no more flash before the mind than can the whole of a mathematical series (cf. Wittgenstein 1953: §187). The invocation of practices, however, is not a move made in the context of the failed strategy, but one that marks a change of strategy.

On a proper interpretation, Wittgenstein rejects the assumption that understanding a rule is an independent mental state which has to be connected to its applications via some mediating process. Instead, he claims that nothing mediates understanding and its applications. There are no explanatory inter-mediaries between understanding a word and making the correct use of it. When one comes to understand the meaning of a word, one acquires the ability to use it correctly. One masters a practice or technique.

This practical reorientation is coupled with Wittgenstein's rejection of the idea that signs are injected with meaning through acts of understanding. He rejects the division of language into 'inorganic' signs and 'organic' understanding:

> It seems that there are *certain definite* mental processes bound up with the working of language, processes through which alone language can function. I mean the processes of understanding and meaning. The signs of our language seem dead without these mental processes; and it might seem that the only function of the signs is to induce such processes, and that these are the things we ought really to be interested in ... We are tempted to think that the action of language consists of two parts; an inorganic part, the handling of signs, and an organic part, which we may call understanding these signs, meaning them, interpreting them, thinking. (Wittgenstein 1958: 3)

Practices are not deployed within the context of the two component picture of language but as a replacement for it. The problem with that picture springs from the distinction it draws between the 'mental state' of understanding and the subsequent use of a word. Once that gap is opened up, nothing can close it.

Instead, understanding the meaning of a word has to be characterised via the practice of using it. Understanding a meaning is a piece of 'know-how', a practical ability. This is anti-reductionist in two senses. First, there is no prospect for a reduction of understanding to causal processes or internal information-carrying states. Secondly, in connecting understanding to prac-tices, the description of the practice cannot be in norm-free terms if meaning is still to be in view.

The ability to understand meaning is a *primitive* ability which cannot be broken down into constitutive parts, but once the 'master thesis' that mental states are free-standing and world-independent states of inner space has been rejected, this should no longer seem mysterious. Meaning can be seen to be a part of the natural history of humans, grounded in our practical abilities. Thus, meaning can be 'naturalised' albeit not in reductionist terms. It is not that reasons are reduced to causes or the space of reasons to the realm of law.

So far I have described understanding linguistic rules that comprise a grasp of meaning. What account of intentional mental states does Wittgenstein offer? Some lessons translate directly from his account of understanding meaning. No account of intentional states that starts from free-standing mental repre-sentations can work. This is a rejection of the master thesis again. Instead, the essence of mental states is their world-directed character, but language does play a key role. In the passage quoted a little earlier, the Wittgensteinian philosopher John McDowell comments: 'Of course I am capable of forming that intention only because I am party to the practices that are constitutive of the relevant concepts' (McDowell 1998b: 315). So as discursive psychology claims, there is a connection between having mental states and possessing a language, but that connection need not be constructionist.

In a later passage from the *Philosophical Investigations* concerning the connection between expectation and what fulfils it Wittgenstein gives a clue as to this connection:

> But it might now be asked: what's it like for him to come?—The door opens, someone walks in, and so on.—What's it like for me to expect him to come?—I walk up and down the room, look at the clock now and then, and so on.—But the one set of events has not the smallest similarity to the other! So how can one use the same words in describing them?—But perhaps I say as I walk up and down: 'I expect he'll come in.'— Now there is a similarity somewhere. But of what kind?!
>  It is in language that an expectation and its fulfilment make contact. (Wittgenstein 1953: §444–5)

Three reinforcing positive suggestions can be derived from these passages. The words that comprise the characteristic expression of a mental state can be converted into a description of its fulfilment condition. Furthermore, mental states are individuated by their fulfilment conditions. Thirdly, the connection between a mental state and its fulfilment mirrors the linguistic connection between the characteristic expression of a state, the description of the state and the description of its fulfilment condition.

The last point, especially, suggests the role of language in a Wittgensteinian account of mental states. In order to be able to think a thought one needs to be able to think what would fulfil it, but this implies that possession of a repertoire of thoughts and mastery of a language go hand in hand. It is not that in speaking a language, or in joining in a conversation, one generally constructs one's thoughts by one's utterances. This point needs some delicacy. Wittgenstein explicitly criticises a picture in which, when one speaks meaningfully, there is a parallel train of thoughts alongside a train of words. The thought or meaning is in the words as expression is carried by musical notes, but it is not that thought can be explained, as social constructionism asserts, through piecemeal social acts. Rather, possession of language enables one to think thoughts that can also be put into words so that one can also think in words if one wishes. It is natural for such linguistic and thus cognitive mastery to become second nature for us.

## Bolton and Hill's alternative use of Wittgenstein

In their book *Mind, Meaning, and Mental Disorder*, the psychologist and philosopher Derek Bolton and the psychiatrist Jonathan Hill attempt a different way to use Wittgensteinian arguments to account for the place of meaning in nature that I will now outline before returning to consider what truth there may be in discursive psychology and cognitivism.

In broad metaphysical terms, Bolton and Hill suggest that the categories of mind and matter as they have been understood since Descartes' time cannot be reconciled without crediting matter with some of the properties previously ascribed only to mind. Likewise, instead of distinguishing between rational reasons and causes—or the space of reasons and the realm of law—they distinguish between intentional and non-intentional causes. This places the hard physical sciences on one side of the divide and the equally hard biological and behavioural sciences on the other. Everyday psychological explanations—folk psychology—are classified alongside and continuously with sciences that invoke the notion of information alongside that of causality. What was useful and appropriate about the distinction between reasons and causes can be captured by the new distinction without incurring its difficulties. Reason explanation is a form of intentional-causal explanation as exemplified in many respectable sciences.

In order for this strategy to work, some account is needed of how intentional causality is appropriate for describing mind and meaning. Bolton and Hill summarise the flow of their argument as follows:

> The first step ... is that explanation of action in terms of meaningful states has predictive power; the second is ... that such explanation is causal; the third is the assumption ... that the brain causally regulates action, all of which can be made compatible on the methodological assumption that the meaning (information) that regulates action is encoded in the brain. (Bolton and Hill 2004: 86)

The idea is as follows. The explanatory power of everyday intentional or 'folk psychological' explanation derives from the causal power of reasons, but the historical division between reasons and causes voiced, for example, by Karl Jaspers (see Chapter 3) puts this claim under threat. If, instead, one distinguishes between intentional and non-intentional causation, folk psychological explanation ceases to be exceptional, and in need of special philosophical explanation, and becomes instead a particular example of a more general phenomenon. This, however, requires some explanation in turn. How is it possible that reasons are a species of intentional causality? Is the information deployed in other intentional-causal sciences, such as biology, of the same order, and explanatory of the meaning that is found in mental health care? The recent philosophical problem is not so much to determine *whether* reasons are causes, but *how* it is possible that reasons are causes.

The solution that Bolton and Hill propose is that the brain encodes meaning. This slogan receives mainly negative characterisation. It is not intended as an attempt to reduce meaning or content to non-intentional terms. Such projects, according to Bolton and Hill, presuppose the fallacious distinction between reasons and causes and attempt to reconcile them by showing that one side is really an instance of the other.

Nor is the slogan a claim on behalf of the idea of Fodor's language of thought hypothesis (discussed in the first section of this chapter). The authors reject representationalist or cognitivist explanations of mental content by invoking the later Wittgenstein's attack on theories based upon static inner states or syntax. They present the following challenge:

> [T]he point is that we can ask of any proposed model of encoding information: 'In what sense is there anything *semantic* here?' (Bolton and Hill 2004: 71)

Following Wittgenstein, they argue that what makes something meaningful is that it plays a role in the guidance of action:

> [W]hat you have to add to, or have instead of, symbol manipulation, in order to achieve intentionality is the regulation of action, that is, meaningful (goal-directed, plastic) interactions with the environment. (Bolton and Hill 2004: 70)

Brain states do not encode meaning by embodying internal syntactic or sentence-like structures but by guiding action in accordance with norms. Clearly, establishing the semantics of neural states will require more than just the claim that they *cause* action. I will return to this point later, but the fundamental connection between meaning and action begins to answer the question of why neural states possess semantics.

This view of the connection between meaning and action is reinforced by a discussion of Wittgenstein's account of rules which they summarise as follows:

> The negative conclusion of Wittgenstein's analysis of rule-following is that the rule is not laid down in advance; the positive implication is that is that it is created in practice. (Bolton and Hill 2004: 127)

Nevertheless, contrary to Wittgenstein's insistence on the impossibility of reducing rules to causal mechanisms, rules do play a *causal* role in the explanation of action according to Bolton and Hill:

> [E]xplanations that invoke meaningful states are effective in prediction: they attribute propensity to follow rules, and hence serve to predict what the agent will do. (Bolton and Hill 2004: 48)

It is this combination of content-laden or intentional and causal powers that is supposed to be explained by the claim that the brain encodes or realises meaning. States of the brain uncontentiously play a causal role in the production of action. But these same states have to be described in information-involving terms if what is to be explained is purposive intentional action as opposed to mere proximal bodily movement. Describing brain states in information-rich terms is appropriate because of the encoding thesis.

The final three chapters of *Mind, Meaning and Mental Disorder* apply a pluralism with respect to the explanation of mental disorder that follows from the continuity amongst the behavioural sciences provided by the notion of intentional causation. With that idea in hand, there is no longer a justification for a strict distinction between meaningful and merely causal symptoms. Symptoms can be both caused and carry meaning if they result from intentional-causal mechanisms. Such mechanisms occur at different levels in the brain's hierarchy: at the level of the personal and the sub-personal. Intentional explanations are appropriate whenever and at whatever level a coherent account of the functioning of intentional-causal mechanisms can be given. Non-intentional causal explanations are appropriate only when there is a breakdown of meaningful relations resulting from brute external factors.

The key idea in these chapters is that illnesses can result from a conflict of the rules which guide an agent's action:

> Humans are physiologically adapted to a narrow range of environmental conditions, but they possess the capacity to devise a wide range of strategies for action, and hence are able to live in very varied environments. The possession of multiple and acquired internalised rules for action, which may be matched to contrasting environmental demands, has therefore been of considerable survival value. However, with the capacity to acquire rules of perception, thought and action, there has arisen the possibility that the operation of intentional-causal processes will not be smooth. In contrast to non-intentional causality the elements of intentional-causal processes ... do not necessarily work in harmony ... If we assume that the efficient function of an intentional causal sequence in a physiological system has evolved over several million years, then the learning of new rules for perceptions and actions over hours, days, months, or even a few years, may seem to be a precarious truncation of the process! (Bolton and Hill 2004: 300)

On the basis of this suggestion, there follows a discussion of schizophrenia, anxiety disorders and personality disorders. It is suggested that each condition may be the meaning-laden result of conflicts between different rules for action. This suggests that the need for brute non-intentional-causal explanation—which seems to preclude meaningful symptoms—may be much diminished.

## Objections to Bolton and Hill

The encoding thesis is supposed to bridge a distinction of kind between, in Jaspers' terms, reasons and causes or, better, between the space of reasons and the realm of law. This, in turn, is supposed to suggest that intentional causation allows of degrees and can apply both to whole people, but also sub-personal elements to shed light on psychopathology and yet more basic intentional-causal sciences such as biology. According to the encoding thesis, intentional contents, such as reasons, are encoded in structures in the brain, which in turn both guide and cause action. However, given the encoding thesis, the claim that the content or semantic properties of brain states—as opposed to their physical properties—is causally active, appears gratuitous.

Bolton and Hill are aware of this objection. Their response is to say that what plays an explanatory role depends on what sort of thing needs to be explained:

> The point is in brief that *if* the goal is explanation and prediction of intentional behaviour (complex organism-environment interactions), *then* the methodological assumption has to be that the agent is regulated by information about the environment, that is, by intentional states, either mental, or encoded in the brain, or both. It is, on the other hand, perfectly possible to do away with intentional concepts, but then only non-intentional behaviour can be predicted, for example, physical movements of the body. (Bolton and Hill 2004: 73)

This response, however, simply reiterates the phenomenon for which the encoding thesis was supposed to be an explanation. It is thus worth examining the encoding thesis in more detail. The thesis is first introduced in the following way:

> At its starkest, the problem [of the contrast between mind and brain] may be expressed by saying that mental states have meaning—carry information—while neural states do not. But, of course, the reply is then simply that this is not true: neural states do carry information. It is axiomatic in the area of overlap between cognitive science and neuroscience that information-processing is implemented by the brain. In brief: neural states encode, and process, information. (Bolton and Hill 2004: 61)

This passage suggests that the encoding thesis is sustained by a view of information processing amongst sub-personal units derived from the cognitive sciences, but it is a mistake to identify the genuinely semantic content that plays a role in guiding and explaining action with the ascriptions of content that are useful in explanations of sub-personal elements of the brain. Taking the familiar question of what the frog's eye tells the frog's brain and the frog itself, McDowell argues that:

> The fact that there is this perfectly intelligible interplay between what we decide we can correctly say, in content-involving terms, about frogs, on the one hand, and the detail of a content-involving (information-processing) account of the inner workings of the parts of frogs, on the other, is no reason to mix the two stories together. In the account of inner workings, one sub-froggy part of a frog transmits information to another: the frog's eye talks to the frog's brain, not to the frog. In the sense in which the frog's eye tells the frog's brain things, nothing tells the frog anything. We may still want to say that the frog gets told things but what does *this* telling is not something in the frog's interior ... Rather, what tells the frog things is the environment, making features of itself apparent to the frog, equipped as it is with frog-perceptual apparatus ...

> Underneath the metaphor of the environment telling the frog things, we have the literal truth that the frog becomes informed of things. Whereas the content-involving truth at the 'sub-personal' level is irreducibly metaphorical. (McDowell 1998b: 349)

The ascription of reasons is tied to making sense of an agent's behaviour in the world. This is the answer to the question Bolton and Hill raise about the semantic status of inner states or structures. Whilst the neurophysiological account of the workings of brains may help itself to the notion of content or, more precisely, information, this is not content in the sense of what is present in the rational structure of reasons.

The latter form of content—which is genuinely semantic—is linked to subjects' experience of the world and the content of reasons concerns worldly states of affairs which are relevant to action. By contrast the information processing model of the brain does not concern world-involving or semantic content. According to McDowell, it is content only in a metaphorical sense, but, less contentiously, one might say that it is an abstraction from, rather than an explanation of, the primary sense of content. Hence, there is a tension when Bolton and Hill say (quoted above): 'the agent is regulated by information about the environment, that is, by intentional states, either mental, or encoded in the brain'. It is one thing to be 'regulated' by the environment when, for example, one reaches towards a kettle one can see. It is quite another to be 'regulated' by the information in the brain. Intentionality or semantics appear only at the level of whole organisms acting for reasons in the world. This is one of the features of mental content that a Wittgensteinian emphasis on the centrality of practice underlies. Despite their criticisms of representationalist and syntactic theories of content such as the language of thought, Bolton and Hill appear to be blind to it at key moments.

The problem is not the claim that reason explanation is causal. It may be that the best way to think of how reasons shed light on action is as a species of causal explanation, but the attempt to explain this, and thus to blur the distinction between the space of reasons and realm of law through the encoding thesis is not successful. The thesis itself prompts two questions for which there is no answer:

- exactly how and according to what rules does the brain encode content? and
- why is it that the content is causal rather than the physical structures that are supposed to carry that content?

The motivation for the encoding thesis appears to be the Wittgensteinian insight that reasons are centrally involved in the guidance of action combined with the empirical claim that the brain is causally responsible for controlling action. It does not follow from this, however, that the brain guides action.

In assuming that it does, Bolton and Hill have not sufficiently left behind the representationalist theory of mind that they criticise.

The only partial success in reconciliation of rationality and causality is also visible in the account of rule following. Bolton and Hill interpret Wittgenstein's critique of explanatory theories of rules as an attack on the idea that the correct use of a sign can be determined in advance by a rule. They conclude instead that correctness in the use of a sign is constructed by ongoing practice, but the problem with this constructivist reading, as set out earlier in this chapter, is that it undermines a central pre-philosophical claim about rules and reasons: that they guide action normatively. They determine those actions that would satisfy them and those which would not in advance. On the Bolton and Hill reading, this normative prescription is replaced by an ongoing causal determination. Whilst such an interpretation of Wittgenstein seems to enable reasons and causes to be tied together, in fact it undermines the very idea of guidance by reason.

This failure to reconcile the rule-guided and the causal also undermines the account of mental disorder in the last part of *Mind, Meaning and Mental Health*. There the idea of merging levels of intentional causality leads to the idea of rule conflict as an explanation for much mental disorder. The strategy helps make the characterisation and explanation of mental disorder philosophically unproblematic. Indeed, it seems a matter of mere good fortune or parenting that in general our rules for action are in harmony and do not lead to disorder, but the complete absence of paradoxicality, in fact suggests that there is something wrong with the account.

Rule conflict appears not only comprehensible, but also highly likely given an appeal to subpersonal rules and content. However, that appeal is illicit unless positive argument is given that internal states have semantic content and can thus serve as reasons. Bolton and Hill claim that the role that inner states play in the guidance of action underpins their content-laden semantic status. Clearly, not all states that merely *produce* or *cause* action are content-laden. Thus, the claim that inner states are reasons *for* and *guide* actions requires further support than the claim that they lead to action. Rule following behaviour must be intentional.

What then justifies this stronger claim? The only plausible answer to this question turns on the role of inner states in a person's overall mental economy, not on atomic facts about the states' causal efficacy. Such support turns, in part, upon the role that the inner states play in the guidance of action, but only in the context of a broader interpretation of the agent which connects the agent to the world. Given this broader interpretative account, rule conflict becomes paradoxical because it requires contravention of the general claim that reasons are rationally structured. Answering the semantic question also provides a general answer to why the rules and reasons that govern behaviour are generally in harmony. They must be because reasons are rationally structured.

What makes Bolton and Hill's account of disorder plausible is the deployment of subpersonal rules that are not yet in harmony, but that turns out to beg the key question they themselves raise: why think of inner states as reasons for actions, rather than mere causes? Without an answer to that question, the methodological pluralism that they espouse appears to be a vacillation between the two sides of the old dichotomy, rather than a confident ability not to have to chose. The question of whether a symptom is a meaningful response to an unusual stimulus or a breakdown of meaningful relations remains as pressing as ever. Do such illnesses lie within the space of reasons or the realm of law? The failure to reconcile the causal and contentful role of inner states in the context of mental disorder reflects their general failure to reconcile reasons and causes through the encoding thesis. Without a satisfactory general reconciliation of the rational and the causal, there can be no sound basis for an answer to these questions.

## The implications of the Wittgensteinian account for cognitivism and discursive psychology

This final subsection will look at the positive consequences of a Wittgensteinian account of meaning for both discursive psychology and for cognitivism. So far in both areas arguments drawn from the later Wittgenstein have been used to criticise discursive psychology and cognitivism. But can anything be salvaged from either account which accords with the positive account of meaning sketched above? I will start with discursive psychology and then make a brief comment about cognitivism.

The second section of this chapter stressed the point that if discursive psychology is a genuine alternative to cognitivism, it must advance a constitutive rather than a merely causal claim about meaning. Meaning has to be constituted, in some sense, in discourse, not just caused by it (as anger might be caused by harsh words). Social constructionism seemed to provide a way to underpin such a constitutive claim. If meanings are constituted in ongoing conversations then they cannot be constituted by factors in the head, but social constructionism is a flawed account of meaning or intentionality. So if not constructionism, what might underpin a constitutive claim and thus underpin a difference between discursive psychology and cognitivism?

A clue lies in the passage quoted earlier:

> In this sense, the psychological is not reducible to or replaceable by explanations in terms of physiology, physics, or any other point of view that does not reveal the structure of meanings existing in the lives of the human group to which the subject of an investigation belongs. (Harré and Gillett 1994: 20)

Constructionism is one reason for denying that the psychological is reducible to states in the head, that no lower level description will capture 'the structure of meanings existing in the lives of the human group'. On the assumption that constructionism is not a coherent approach to mind and meaning, however, what other reason might there be for denying the reduction to states within the head?

One reason has already been articulated in this chapter. If Wittgenstein's rejection of what McDowell calls the 'master thesis', that the mind is populated with items that have to be interpreted in order to relate to the world, is correct and if there are principled reasons why normative notions of the space of reasons cannot be reduced to the non-normative realm of law, then one version of discursive psychology's constitutive claim is justified. On a Wittgensteinian account, neither meaning nor mental content can be reduced to free-standing states in the head as cognitivism assumes.

There is, however, another family of approaches within American philosophy of mind and language, which could also underpin discursive psychology. Borrowing from the accounts proposed by philosophers such as Daniel Dennett and Donald Davidson, discursive psychology could take its subject matter to be the rational pattern in human speech and action, a pattern that has no echo in underlying physical and neurological descriptions.

Both Davidson and Dennett argue that the ascription of meanings and mental states is essentially tied to an interpretative strategy: the Radical Interpretation and the Intentional Stance, respectively (Davidson 1984: 207–25; Dennett 1987: 13–35). By describing the strategy, they provide insight into the nature of the states—mental states and meanings—it describes. Dennett compares and contrasts the Intentional Stance to two other strategies: the 'Physical Stance' and the 'Design Stance'. The former is based on physical laws; the latter on the assumption that a system will behave as it is designed to. The Intentional Stance, in turn, is based on predicting that a system will behave in accordance with the dictates of rationality applied in context.

Davidson approaches mind and meaning by considering the conditions of possibility of making sense of the speech and action of others from scratch: the Radical Interpretation of a marooned anthropologist. Arguing that the ascriptions of beliefs and of meanings (to native speech) form an interdependent whole with only one source of evidence (correlations between utterances and worldly features), he argues that interpretation requires a Principle of Charity to constrain it. The thought experiment, however, also captures our own epistemic predicament because the justification for knowledge of the meaning of terms in one's own native language terminates in Radical Interpretation of the surrounding community. Thus, both Dennett and Davidson argue that minds and meanings both form essentially rational patterns, and are essentially tied to the public realm of speech and action because of their essential connection to an interpretative stance. It is of the essence of mind to be detectable from a third person point of view. That claim marks a contrast with cognitivism where that connection is merely contingent.

The contrast is more pronounced if there is also reason to think that the pattern of meanings in the lives of humans is not reproduced as a physiological pattern within their skulls. Such an isomorphism would suggest a possible reconciliation of cognitivist and discursive approaches with distinct, but equivalent, subject matters. An argument for this stronger contrast is, however, already implicit in the discussion of Wittgenstein above. No internal physiological state can have the normative properties of meaning. Davidson adds to this Wittgensteinian claim a parallel argument based more closely on rationality than normativity. He claims that any such parallelism would require that rational connections could be mapped onto a nomological pattern, but as they answer to distinct constitutive principles this is highly unlikely. The rational pattern of the space of reasons would have somehow to be captured in a pattern of neurological laws and, thus, what makes one belief rational in the light of others would have to be captured using, for example, some statistical laws of association. The kind of relations available in the realm of law, however, look to be the wrong sort to capture the underlying notion of a rational connection in the space of reasons (see also McDowell 1998b: 325–40)

There is, then, a different way of underpinning the constitutive claim needed to distinguish a discursive turn from a form of cognitivism, which admits that social factors can cause mental effects. The constitutive claim can be underpinned by a view of meaning that ties it to a rational pattern in human lives without the need to argue, in agreement with the concomitant crudity of the constructionist claim, that the pattern is constructed *de novo* in ongoing judgement.

A non-constructionist version of the discursive approach also subscribes to a different version of naturalism. I suggested at the start of the chapter that cognitivism is a form of reductionist naturalism because it aims to fit minds and meanings into nature by reducing the mind to a mechanism characterized in information-processing terms. I suggested in the second section that constructionist versions of discursive psychology also subscribe to a form of reductionist naturalism, albeit not a reduction to states in the head. They take the notion of meaning, especially its normative properties, to be problematic and attempt to reconstruct them from something more basic and less philosophically puzzling. Both a Wittgensteinian approach to meaning outlined above and also Dennett and Davidson's 'stance stance' approach to mind-meaning also deserve to be called forms of naturalism. They aim to show how minds and meanings fit unproblematically into nature, but they attempt no reduction. Connections are made to practices, and to interpretation and rationality, respectively, but no concept is taken to be more basic. Thus, properly understood, discursive psychology can be taken to contrast with reductionist naturalism after all.

Whilst a view of discursive psychology can be reconstructed that escapes a Wittgensteinian critique, things are more difficult in the case of cognitivist accounts of meaning. The problem in this case is that cognitivism is committed to claims that run directly counter to the Wittgensteinian idea that the basic unit of meaning is not an inner mental representation, but the life of the whole person. Nevertheless, one aspect of cognitivism does deserve further thought. What can be made of the functional dependence diagrams, such as Ellis' model of understanding meaning?

Such models can be interpreted in either of two ways. They can be seen as bottom-up explanations of human thought that deploy a basic notion of information manipulated by different sub-personal systems. Alternatively, they can be seen as an abstraction from the notion of meaning or content that depends on the action—the navigation about the world—of whole persons. On this latter interpretation, information is not explanatorily basic. It does not explain meaning or content, but presupposes it. Only the latter view is consistent with the Wittgensteinian critique developed in this chapter, but it does provide a way to interpret the functional dependence diagrams found in cognitivist psychiatry. They serve as a kind of shorthand for and partial explanation of human linguistic abilities. They are abstractions from, rather than explanations of, normal human abilities, but they can shed light on the way complex linguistic abilities, which are normally found together are co-related.

## 4. Conclusions

As Chapter 3 outlined, Karl Jaspers stressed the importance, alongside causal explanation, of understanding the experience and thought processes of sufferers of mental illness. Meaning is thus central to mental health care, but this raises a key question: what is the relation between meaningful phenomena and other natural facts and events? How is meaning—or the content of mental states—a part of nature? How do reasons relate to causes or the space of reasons to the realm of law?

Two main theoretical approaches within mental health care suggest different answers to this question. According to cognitivist approaches, meaning is to be explained on the basis of information-processing computers. Reasons are a species of causes and intentionality or semantics is explained as an essentially causal notion. According to constructionist forms of discursive psychology, meaning is the ongoing product of conversations. Although these are contrasting approaches, they share a common aim: that of explaining meaning or intentionality in more basic non-meaning-presupposing terms. Such reductionism, however, faces grave objections.

A third option, set out recently by Bolton and Hill, attempts to reconcile reasons and causes by distinguishing, instead, between intentional and non-intentional causation. This is, in turn, further characterised through the slogan that the brain encodes meaning. The problem with their solution, however, is not the idea that reasons can be causes—which might be accepted as the best account of action explanation—but rather the idea that that claim is explained through the slogan that brains encode meaning. With that slogan in play, the question of *how* the brain encodes content and why it is the content that is causal, rather than the physical structures that are supposed to carry that content, both become pressing.

The alternative is to embrace meaning and intentionality as features of the world which are natural in their own right. This non-reductive or relaxed naturalism has two aspects. Human subjects possess abilities that, through suitable education and training, can be moulded into an appreciation of meanings. It is a natural feature of human beings that we can take part in linguistic and other meaning-laden practices that underpin our mindedness. We can make judgements about what others mean and can, in turn, judge how to use language appropriately. This ability cannot be reduced to mere mechanisms.

This view also includes the claim that the world itself contains not just those features that can be explained using the nomological causal explanations of the realm of law, but also the meaning-laden phenomena of the space of reasons. Psychiatry needs therefore to embrace an augmented sense of nature or the world, a relaxed form of naturalism. The next chapter will add to considerations of Chapters 1 and 2 that such an enlarged sense of nature should also include values.

# Part III

# **Facts**

## Chapter 5

# The validity of psychiatric classification

## Plan of the chapter

This chapter will consider the question: 'Is psychiatric classification valid?' It will explore the presuppositions that make that question pressing for psychiatry, outline two discussions about the nature of psychiatric classification that have a bearing on validity and examine some of the resources for assessing it drawn from the philosophy of science.

Classification is fundamental to all sciences. It lies at the heart of any kind of conceptual judgement, which is a matter of placing individual phenomena into patterns of general kinds. It also lies at the heart of prediction and explanation. If new phenomena are judged to be of the same kind as those previously encountered, then they can be expected to behave in relevantly similar respects both prospectively (prediction) and retrospectively (explanation).

Classifications can, of course, come in different forms. There can be groupings into rigid and mutually exclusive kinds, groupings on the basis of a number of possibly overlapping factors and relations based on continuously varying mathematical quantities. Of any of these varieties of classification it is tempting to ask: is it a *natural* classification, a classification that tracks real, objective underlying similarities in nature, or is it, instead, an imposed classification that may or may not be useful for us, but expresses *our* interests, rather than the shape of the world?

In psychiatry, this question is particularly vivid. It is expressed in concerns about the validity of psychiatric classification and diagnosis. The anti-psychiatry movement, discussed in Chapter 1, argues that psychiatric classifications are not reflections of genuine medical conditions at all, but are instead reflections of social prescriptions and values. Even some of those who do not subscribe to such an extreme view argue that psychiatry differs from physics and engineering by containing an essentially evaluative aspect. Nevertheless, it is then a further question to ask what follows for the objectivity of psychiatry if this is true. Is an objective medical model based on a descriptivist account of illness a necessary component of any account that grants psychiatry scientific status? Is there only one kind of objectivity at work here?

Even amongst psychiatrists completely opposed to the anti-psychiatry movement, the validity of psychiatric diagnosis is a central concern. It is, for example, flagged in Chapter 1 of *A Research Agenda for DSM-V* (Kupfer *et al.* 2002). Whilst the move to operationalised definitions has increased the reliability of DSM-III and IV, it does not necessarily ensure the underlying validity of the classifications. Among specific issues raised for the development of DSM-V is whether classification should be based on aetiological factors or prognosis:

> [S]hould it be argued that—although etiological based diagnosis is the ultimate goal of psychiatric nosology—this is currently impractical and the time-honoured practical validators—course, outcome, response to treatment, etc.—should continue to be used …? (Kupfer *et al.* 2002: 8–9)

The authors go on to question whether classification should be based on dimensions instead of categories, and whether mental illnesses can be construed as discrete entities or not. However, the main concern is whether the recent emphasis on psychiatric reliability should now be replaced by concern with validity.

The first section of this chapter starts by examining the broader connection between the debate about values and the analysis discussed in Chapter 1 and the validity of psychiatric classification. It summarises Hempel's advice about psychiatric classification, and its connections to both reliability and validity. Next, it examines the nature of validity in more detail, and the connection between validity and the presence of values in psychiatric classification. I argue that even if psychiatric classification is value-laden that need not undermine its validity. The assumption that it must is based on a questionable neo-Humean view of values.

The second section introduces two further 'internal' complications. The first is criticism of the design of psychiatric classification by Kendell and Jablensky. The second is the call for the inclusion of a narrative element in a model of comprehensive psychiatric diagnosis. This raises issues for validity because, in a nutshell, most models of validity are nomothetic, but narrative elements are idiographic.

The third section outlines some tools from the philosophy of science for assessing these issues. By discussing tests of validity drawn from the philosophy of science, I argue first that there is no independent theory neutral test of psychiatric validity. Nothing can replace the element of clinical judgement in assessing the evidence for a taxonomy. Secondly, narrative elements in diagnosis can be assessed for validity, but only using the standard of judgements of rational plausibility.

## 1. **Facts, values and psychiatric validity**

### Hempel's contribution to the debate about psychiatric classification

Hempel was one of the developers of the Logical Empiricist picture of science, which was influential in the middle period of the 20th century. In 1959 he was invited by the American Psychological Association to present a paper at a conference of psychiatrists in order to aid the development of a more scientific system of classification.

Despite the efforts of Emil Kraepelin and others in the early years of the 20th century, the classification of psychiatric disorders had been chaotic up to the Second World War. Immediately on its foundation in 1945, the World Health Organisation (WHO) set about establishing an International Classification of Diseases (ICD) as an essential tool for its work. Most chapters of the classification, those dealing with bodily disorders, were well received and readily adopted around the world. The psychiatric section alone proved problematic, with most countries, indeed most psychiatric institutions, continuing to operate with their own systems.

The WHO commissioned the British psychiatrist, Erwin Stengel, to investigate why this had happened and to propose a basis for a classification that would be more widely acceptable. It was in this connection that the conference was set up, at which Hempel, as a philosopher of science, was invited to speak. Stengel chaired Hempel's session and some of Hempel's ideas provided the basis for his report to the WHO.

In fact, the key change Stengel proposed was based on an intervention by the UK psychiatrist Sir Aubrey Lewis. The change was to abandon attempts at a classification based on theories of the causes of mental disorder (essentially because such theories were premature) and to rely, instead, on what could be directly observed: that is, symptoms. ICD-8 consequently appeared and was widely adopted. The present version, ICD-10, and, indirectly, DSM-IV, are both derived from ICD-8 and retain its essential basis in symptoms. It is interesting to note that this is not a key moral in Hempel's paper. It instead stresses the eventual goal of theoretically-rather than observationally-based classifications. Arguably, however, psychiatry had not and still has not reached that stage of development. (For a full account of the relationship between Hempel's paper, Lewis' intervention and Stengel's conclusions see (Fulford *et al.* 2006: 320–41).)

There was a parallel influence from within American psychiatry that shaped the writing of DSM-III. Whilst DSM-I and DSM-II had drawn heavily on psychoanalytic theoretical terms, the committee charged with drawing up DSM-III drew on the work of a group of psychiatrists from Washington University of St Louis. Responding in part to research that had revealed significant differences in diagnostic practices between different psychiatrists, the 'St Louis group', led by John Feighner, published operationalised criteria for psychiatric diagnosis. The DSM-III task force replaced reference to Freudian aetiological theory with more observational criteria. The task force leader, Robert Spitzer, later reported: 'With its intellectual roots in St Louis instead of Vienna, and with its intellectual inspiration drawn from Kraepelin, not Freud, the task force was viewed from the outset as unsympathetic to the interests of those whose theory and practice derived from the psychoanalytic tradition' (Bayer and Spitzer 1985: 188, quoted in Shorter 1997: 301–2).

In his paper, Hempel claims that scientific classifications or taxonomies must meet two requirements:

> Broadly speaking, the vocabulary of science has two basic functions: first, to permit an adequate *description* of the things and events that are the objects of scientific investigation; second, to permit the establishment of general laws or theories by means of which particular events may be *explained* and *predicted* and thus *scientifically understood*; for to understand a phenomenon scientifically is to show that it occurs in accordance with general laws or theoretical principles. (Hempel 1994: 317)

Hempel argues that the terms employed in classifications should have clear, public criteria of application and they should lend themselves to the formulation of general laws, which reflect natural uniformities. To put this in medical terms, these aims correspond to the aims of *reliability* and *validity*. Both of these requirements reflect different aspects of the more general requirement that scientific taxonomies should be objective.

Hempel suggests that there is usually a change in the balance between how these requirements are met during the development and maturation of scientific research programmes or disciplines:

> In fact ... the development of a scientific discipline may often be said to proceed from an initial 'natural history' stage, which primarily seeks to describe the phenomena under study and to establish simple empirical generalisations concerning them, to subsequent more and more theoretical stages ... (Hempel 1994: 317)

Given this transition, Hempel should not be interpreted as advocating that psychiatry remains at the stage of natural history. He does not lobby for observational classifications. Nevertheless, meeting the requirement of reliability is important. It plays a key role in his account of what scientific objectivity involves:

> Science aims at knowledge that is *objective* in the sense of being intersubjectively certifiable, independently of individual opinion or preference, on the basis of data obtainable by suitable experiments or observations. This requires that the terms used in formulating scientific statements have clearly specified meanings and be understood in the same sense by all those who use them. (Hempel 1994: 318)

To take the aim of reliability first. This is defined as the degree of agreement between users of a classification. Two main kinds of reliability are usually recognised. *Inter-observer* or *inter-rater* reliability is the extent to which two or more observers agree about the classification (diagnosis in the medical case) of a given case on a given occasion. *Test–retest* reliability is the degree of agreement by a given observer in his or her classification of a given case over a period of time (but see also Millon *et al.* 1999: 13–14 for others.)

In the context of this aim—the reliability of classifications—Hempel discusses, with approval, the use of operational definitions (following Bridgman's book *The Logic of Modern Physics* 1927), although he emphasises that in psychiatry the kind of measurement operations in terms of which concepts would be defined would have to be construed loosely.

However, this concern with reliability and operationalised definitions is balanced in Hempel by another aim of classification: validity. Hempel introduces this idea as follows:

> But clear and objective criteria of application are not enough; to be scientifically useful a concept must lend itself to the formulation of general laws or theoretical principles which reflect uniformities in the subject matter under study and which thus provide a basis for explanations, prediction, and generally scientific understanding. This aspect of a set of scientific concepts will be called its *systematic import*, for it represents the contribution the concepts make to the systematization of knowledge in the given field by means of laws and theories. The requirement of systematic import applies, in particular, also to the concepts that determine scientific classifications. Indeed, the familiar vague distinction between *natural* and *artificial* classifications may well be explicated as referring to the difference between classifications that are

scientifically fruitful and those that are not ... It is understandable that a classification of this sort should be viewed as somehow having objective existence in nature, as 'carving nature at the joints', in contradistinction to artificial classifications ... (Hempel 1994: 322–4)

I will discuss this aim further shortly, but it will be helpful, first, to introduce Hempel's comments about the consequences for psychiatric classifications of the presence of values:

In the interest of the objective, it may be worth considering whether, or to what extent, criteria with valuational overtones are used in the specification of psychiatric concepts ... Such notions as inadequacy of response, inadaptability, ineptness, and poor judgement clearly have valuational aspects, and it is to be expected that their use in concrete cases will be influenced by the idiosyncrasies of the investigator. This will reduce the reliability of these concepts and of those for which they serve as partial criteria of application. (Hempel 1994: 322)

Hempel's discussion of the 'valuational' aspect of psychiatric classification suggests an important connection to the 'values in' versus 'values out' debate discussed in Chapter 1 between value-theorists and descriptivists. He suggests that values threaten to undermine the objectivity of psychiatric classification. Why is that?

The main argument concerns the reliability of classification and the threat to that of evaluative elements. The idea is that, because different people make different value judgements, then if classifications require value judgements, those classifications will lack reliability.

However, as the discussion in Chapter 1 suggested, there is a potentially direct route between values and a more fundamental lack of objectivity, corresponding to validity, which does not turn on reliability. On the direct route, the presence of values in a classification is enough in itself to show that the classification lacks validity. One way to explain this is to consider an everyday classification that depends on human interests and values.

Consider the example of herbs. These are defined by the *Concise Oxford Dictionary* both as a kind of 'plant of which the stem is not woody or persistent, and which dies down to ground after flowering', but also a kind of 'plant of which leaves etc. are used for food, medicine, scent, flavour etc.' (I will ignore the fact that these are quite distinct definitions, which need not even be extensionally equivalent.) The latter is a functional definition that depends on human culinary practice. It unites a number of different plants, which might have no non-disjunctive biologically necessary and sufficient conditions. If a new plant were discovered, a full description of its biological properties would not determine whether or not it were a herb.

Classifications which express human interests can possess *reliability* (both test–retest and *inter-rater*). Given the definition of herb, there is no reason to doubt the reliability of the classification of items into herbs and non-herbs. (There will, of course, be some grey areas about little used herbs.) However, whilst reliability may be evidence for the second classificatory virtue it does not strictly imply that the classification also possesses *validity*. Can classifications that reflect human values be valid? The question is important because much debate inspired by the anti-psychiatry movement turns on doubts about whether psychiatric classifications reflect *real* as opposed *artefactual* distinctions.

Whether or not the distinction between herbs and non-herbs is valid or not depends on the meaning of validity:

> The word 'valid' is derived from the Latin *validus*, meaning strong, and it is defined as 'well-founded and applicable; sound and to the point; against which no objection can fairly be brought' (Shorter Oxford Dictionary 1978). There is no single, agreed upon meaning of validity in science, although it is generally accepted that the concept addresses 'the nature of reality' (Kerlinger 1973: 456–476) and that its definition is an 'epistemological and philosophical problem, not simply a question of measurement' (Galtung 1969: 121). (Kendell and Jablensky 2003: 5)

In psychological and psychiatric literature at least four kinds of validity are distinguished (in fact, there are others such as concurrent validity):

- *Face validity*: the extent to which a classification appears to be of relevant features, which has consequences for the acceptability of tests to test users and subjects (Rust and Golombok 1989: 78).

- *Construct validity*: roughly, the extent to which it relates to underlying theory. Kendell articulates this thus: 'the demonstration that aspects of psychopathology which can be measured objectively ... do in fact occur in the presence of diagnoses which assume their presence and not in the presence of those which assume their absence' (Kendell 1975b: 40). Anastasi says it is 'the extent to which the test may be said to measure a theoretical construct or trait' (Anastasi 1968: 114).

- *Predictive validity*: the extent to which the classification allows us to predict future properties.

- *Content validity*: 'the demonstration that the defining characteristics of a given disorder are indeed enquired into and elicited before that diagnosis is made' (Kendell 1975b: 40).

The chemical Periodic Table, for example, has a high degree of validity in all these respects. It is *prima facie* relevant (face validity), it is strongly related to underlying theory (the explanation of chemical properties based on electron study), it has high predictive validity (to the extent of anticipating the existence of new elements) and it relies on a set of distinctions based on the *essential* features of elements.

These sub-species of validity, however, do not capture a further, perhaps inchoate, understanding of it. Like reliability, the sub-species have the virtue that they can be, at least partially, measured or assessed. But, to take one example, the fact that a newly devised disease concept reflects a well-established physiological theory and thus possesses construct validity does not establish that the concept corresponds to a genuine judgement-independent entity or type. The theory as a whole may, after all, be wrong. This suggests a further, more general, sense of validity having to do with getting things right. It is hinted at in this quotation:

> Undoubtedly the most important question to be asked about any psychological test concerns its validity, i.e., the degree to which the test actually measures what it purports to measure. Validity provides a direct check on how well the test fulfils its function. (Anastasi 1968: 28)

> The validity of a test concerns what the test measures and how well it does so. (Anastasi 1968: 99)

The more general underlying idea of validity is, however, more difficult both to measure and to explain further. Anastasi goes on to say: 'Fundamentally, all procedures for determining test validity are concerned with relationships between performance on the test and other independently observable facts ...' (Anastasi 1968: 99). She goes on to describe the sub-species of validity in a way that emphasises how *they can* be measured, but as a result plays down the idea that the validity of a test comprises *its actually* measuring what it purports to measure. (In effect this blurs reliability and validity.)

In the case of a classification, its validity in this deeper sense depends on whether it actually describes *genuine underlying* differences. In his discussion of psychiatry, Hempel employs the well worn philosophical phrase by saying that a fruitful classification 'carves nature at its joints' (Hempel 1994: 324). What exactly does this phrase mean? What sense can be applied to that phrase that does not simply help itself to the content of one of our classifications of nature. This point can be emphasised by asking from what perspective can the claim be made? It seems to require stepping outside our classifications to say of them that they line up with real divisions in nature, but how is that even notionally possible? How are the 'real divisions' specified without using another classification whose own naturalness will then be open to question. The difficulty of finding a way to *express* the claim threatens to undermine the idea that there is a genuine claim to make here.

I will consider two characterisations of validity that can be drawn from philosophical work: first a sense based on the idea of cognitive command, which was outlined in Chapter 2, which the herb classification passes, and then one based on mind-independence as discussed by the philosopher, John McDowell, which it fails. The latter, I suggest, influences assessment of the claims of anti-psychiatry.

## Values and two underlying senses of validity

I will turn first to one way of connecting reliability and validity using an idea of the philosopher and metaphysician Crispin Wright. My aim is not to explore this idea in any length, but to use it to draw out an assumption about the nature of psychiatric classification that impacts on anti-psychiatry.

In a book that explores a number of tests for the realism of a discourse Wright proposes one called *cognitive command*:

> It is *a priori* that differences of opinion formulated within the discourse, unless excusable as a result of vagueness in a disputed statement, or in the standards of acceptability, or variation in personal evidence thresholds, so to speak, will involve something which may properly be regarded as a cognitive shortcoming. (Wright 1992: 144)

He gives comedy as an example of something that fails this test. If two people disagree about whether a joke is funny neither, he suggests, need have made a mistake. They may simply have a different taste or sense of humour. For this reason, Wright suggests, one should not be a 'comic realist'.

This test can be used to define one sense of objectivity or validity:

◆ A classificatory judgement is valid if it passes the test of cognitive command.

It is *a priori* that differences in its application imply at least one mistake. Given actual levels of disagreement about what is funny, comedy lacks, in medical terms, *inter-rater* reliability. However, because that disagreement need not imply that any mistake has been made, comedy also fails to have validity in this sense. By contrast, the judgement that something is a herb, although expressive of human interests, passes this test. If two people disagree on whether a herb is used in cooking then, vagueness aside, at least one must have made a mistake. Thus, such judgement or classification possesses this sense of validity.

Note that it might be possible that careful schooling or perhaps brain washing would ensure that everyone did, *as a matter of fact*, agree about the comic quality of jokes without this in any sense increasing the factuality of such judgements. (In a similar vein one can imagine that sufficiently robust policing of the 'profession' of astrology might ensure the reliability (in the medical sense) of astrological description and prediction without increasing its effectiveness (or 'reliability' in the everyday sense).) This is why cognitive command is characterised as an *a priori* claim about the possibility of disagreement.

With this idea in place and with anti-psychiatry in mind, it is intuitive to think that failure of cognitive command corresponds to judgements which are expressive of *values* (evaluations, rather than descriptions). This corresponds to a subset of classifications that reflect human interests: those that also reflect more specifically values. Such kinds appear to fail to possess the sense of validity just defined.

There are, however, some complications to this intuitive view that failure of cognitive command corresponds to the presence of values. Thinking about these will lead me to discuss (and reject) a second sense of validity that will shed light on the nature of psychiatric classification:

- Unless failure of cognitive command is taken to define evaluations (Fulford, e.g., sometimes seems to (Fulford 1989: 48; 1991: 86–8; but see also 2000: 91)) then a further argument is needed that only value judgements fail the test. Without that further argument, it is not clear that the presence of values is *necessary* for judgement to fail the test.

- An argument is also needed to show that judgements of values do fail cognitive command. Take judgements of moral value. Both those who subscribe to a principles approach (e.g. Kantianism) to underpin moral judgement and those who adopt the particularist view of moral judgements outlined in Chapter 2 can argue that if two people disagree about a judgement then at least one of them must have made a mistake either in applying moral principles or perceiving moral features of the world. In other words, it is not clear that the presence of values is *sufficient* for judgement to fail the test. I will return shortly to one source of hostility to this thought.

The intuitive view sheds light on the connection between the presence of normative concepts and anti-psychiatry. As described in Chapter 1, the main argument deployed by Szasz in his paper 'The myth of mental illness' is that mental illnesses differ from physical illnesses in a crucial respect. Whereas physical health and ill health can, according to Szasz, be defined in purely anatomical and physiological terms, mental ill health has to be defined in terms of psychosocial, ethical and legal concepts. Thus, it is 'logically absurd' to expect that medical interventions will help. This is not to say that the social and psychological occurrences which are normally labelled as mental illnesses do not themselves exist. They do, but this does not imply that they are constitutive of illness. The position he outlines: 'stands in sharp opposition to the currently prevalent position, according to which psychiatrists treat mental diseases, which are just as "real" and "objective" as bodily diseases' (Szasz 1972: 19).

I wish to focus on the view that mental illness lacks objectivity because it is defined in psycho-social, ethical and legal concepts. Why would this follow? It would follow on the joint assumption that such concepts are essentially evaluative *and* that values are not parts of the world. The presence of values alone does not imply a failure of cognitive command. An Aristotelian can argue that values are a feature of the world, as outlined in the discussion of moral particularism in Chapter 2. If so, then disagreements between subjects would imply a mistake.

What is necessary, in addition to the presence of values, to undermine the cognitive command of a classification is the further assumption that I will call a 'neo-Humean' view of the place of values in nature. On this view, values are not real features of the world, but depend instead on subjective human reactions or sentiments. With this assumption in place then even if subjects were to agree on value judgements such that they possessed reliability, that would not imply that they had cognitive command. This is because *had* there been disagreement (about the implicit values) this need *not* imply any mistake. (Even Fulford—no anti-psychiatrist—stresses the idea that disagreement in psychiatric diagnosis is explained by reasonable disagreement on underlying implicit values: 'most people most of the time use the term "bad" of apples with brown skins. (But) (t)hey don't *have* to do so' (Fulford 1991: 86).) This thought, whilst plausible, is, however, just an assumption. That assumption can in turn be used to characterise a further sense of validity (see below), but the assumption of neo-Humeanism, once highlighted, can also be called into question.

Neo-Humeanism adds to the (plausible) semantic thesis that value judgements cannot be explained in non-value judgement terms (one cannot derive an *ought* from an *is*) a (dubious) metaphysical thesis that values are not found in nature but only in us. Values are *projected* onto the world rather than found in it. McDowell describes neo-Humeanism thus:

> According to the sort of outlook I mean, reality is exhausted by the natural world, in the sense of the world as the natural sciences are capable of revealing to us. Part of the truth in the idea that science disenchants nature is that science is committed to a dehumanized stance for investigation; that is taken to be a matter of conforming to a metaphysical insight into the character of reality as such ... Any candidate feature of reality that science cannot capture is downgraded as a projection, a result of mind's interaction with the rest of nature. (McDowell 1998b: 175)

The idea is that the world or nature comprises only those features described by natural science (by a basic physics and what can be reduced to it). What cannot be so reduced is not a genuine feature of the world (see Fodor 1987: 97). This view of nature also underpins essentialist views of natural kinds in which the world individuates itself independently of what we know about it. McDowell further characterises it thus:

> A genuine fact must be a matter of the way things are in themselves, utterly independently of us. So a genuinely true judgement must be, at least potentially, an exercise of pure thought; if human nature is necessarily implicated in the very formation of the judgement, that precludes our thinking of the corresponding fact as properly independent of us, and hence as a proper fact at all. (McDowell 1998b: 254)

As well as underpinning the application of cognitive command to value judgement, this can also be used to characterise a further inchoate sense of validity (which, I think, is an assumption of both anti-psychiatry and biologically-minded responses to it alike).

- ◆ A classificatory judgement is valid if it can be characterised using the resources only of a dehumanised natural scientific standpoint, fully independent of human interests.

I left hanging the question of whether the distinction between herbs and non-herbs—a distinction that reflects human culinary tastes and interests—was valid. Although judgements about herbs pass Wright's cognitive command test—and thus we might say were valid in that sense—they lack validity in this different sense, which reflects a neo-Humean view of nature. If neo-Humeanism were a true account of nature and if validity is a measure only of what belongs in nature so construed, then judgements about herbs lack validity.

Despite the plausibility (the face validity!) of this sense of validity and the role, I suggest, it plays in debates about anti-psychiatry it is based on a contentious metaphysical assumption. McDowell raises a number of arguments against it. One problem, described in Chapter 2, is this (McDowell 1998b: 157–60). A projectivist account of, say, moral judgement requires that one can give an account of the subjective response to non-moral features in the world, which is then projected onto the world to give the appearance of moral properties. It is far from clear, however, that that *response* can be characterised in terms that do not *presuppose* the idea that worldly events have moral properties. (As an illustration, McDowell argues that amusement cannot be characterised except in terms of finding some things comic and, thus, cannot *explain* the idea of things being comic.)

A further consideration turns on how features that are apparently worldly, but depend on subjects having a particular perspective (e.g. secondary qualities like colour or taste) can be explained without taking up that perspective (McDowell 1998b: 112–30). Only by adopting such a perspective, McDowell argues, can one make sense of the property concerned and this places principled limits on the explanatory potential of the 'view from nowhere' presupposed by neo-Humeanism.

There is also a more general argument against such mind-independence based on Wittgenstein's account of making judgements in accord with a rule. In the *Philosophical Investigations*, Wittgenstein attacks a Platonist account of our conceptual structure in which correct judgement depends on latching onto an extra-human order (Wittgenstein 1953). He characterises the picture he attacks as one in which the application of a rule consists in going over in bolder pencil moves which have, in a mysterious sense, already been made. As McDowell explains, this applies to empirical judgement in this way:

> We can find this picture [i.e. one where a genuinely true judgement must be, at least potentially, an exercise of pure thought] of genuine truth compelling only if we either forget that truth-bearers are such only because they are meaningful, or suppose that meanings take care of themselves, needing, as it were, no help from us. This latter supposition is the one that is relevant to our concerns. If we make it, we can let the judging subject in our picture of true judgement shrink to a locus of pure thought, while the fact that judging is a human activity fades into insignificance...
>
> When we say 'Diamonds are hard' is true if and only if diamonds are hard, we are just as much involved on the right-hand side as the reflections on rule-following tell us we are. There is a standing temptation to miss this obvious truth, and to suppose that the right-hand side somehow presents us with a possible fact, pictured as a unconceptualised configuration of things in themselves. (McDowell 1998b: 254–5)

McDowell's argument is that *nothing* can occupy the extreme objective end of a scale of objectivity cashed out in terms of mind-independence. The very idea of applying concepts in judgement presupposes a subject who finds it natural to make judgements in a particular way, to find particular ways of going on natural. Thus, despite its initial plausibility, nothing could possess validity in the second sense described above. To the extent to which the debate between anti-psychiatrists and biologically-minded defenders of psychiatry presupposes a neo-Humean view of nature, that debate is misguided.

The alternative picture of nature that McDowell sketches is one of a world containing features whose understanding and detection require the possession of certain conceptual abilities. Only those, for example, with a suitable moral outlook can be responsive to the moral demands which the world makes on us, but these demands are, nevertheless, genuine features of the external world. They are not merely projections onto it. The world contains features whose conceptualisation requires a subject to have particular interests, abilities and even perceptual sensitivities. If this alternative to neo-Humeanism is coherent, then there can be no swift argument from the dependence of a property on human interests to its not being valid. Thus, if psychiatric classification does involve kinds which reflect human interests, that does not impugn its ability to describe real features of the world.

This is not to argue that psychiatric classification is valid even if it contains putatively evaluative elements. The argument is more modest. Contrary to what both Hempel and Szasz imply, the presence of values would not imply a lack of validity, but, of course, if psychiatric classification is on the wrong lines for some other reason, then it will fail of validity. How, then, can that issue be addressed? The next section will outline two specific further complications and the third section examine arguments from the philosophy of science.

## 2. **Two complications for psychiatric classification**

In this short section, I will highlight two more recent developments in psychiatry which specifically raise issues for the validity of its taxonomy. The first is a family of criticisms of the current approach to psychiatric classification from within scientific psychiatry. The second is the recent suggestion from within the World Psychiatric Association that diagnosis should be based not only on a general criterial approach but also on a person specific narrative account. Using the terminology of Windelband from Chapter 3, it adds an 'idiographic', individualised element to the law-like or 'nomothetic' approach exemplified in the ICD-10 and DSM-IV schema. The first confronts the issue of validity head on. The second has indirect consequences for validity.

### Kendell and Jablensky and the 'disease entity' assumption

In addition to a general scepticism, prompted by anti-psychiatry, about psychiatric taxonomy, based on the presence of values, there are also more specific arguments against its validity framed from within psychiatry. These sometimes take the form of favouring a different kind of classification such as one based on ideal types or on individual symptoms, rather than whole syndromes, or on continuously varying dimensions, rather than discrete entities.

One example of such internal criticism is provided by Robert Kendell and Assen Jablensky in their paper 'Distinguishing between the validity and utility of psychiatric diagnoses'. They discuss what they take to be an 'insidious reification' of diseases or syndromes:

> Thoughtful clinicians have long been aware that diagnostic categories are simply concepts, justified only by whether they provide a useful framework for organizing and explaining the complexity of clinical experience in order to derive inferences about outcome and to guide decisions about treatment. Unfortunately, once a diagnostic concept such as schizophrenia or Gulf War syndrome has come into general use, it tends to become reified. That is people too easily assume that it is an entity of some kind that can be invoked to explain the patient's symptoms and whose validity need not be questioned. (Kendell and Jablensky 2003: 5)

This passage raises the following concern. Are the diseases picked out in psychiatric classifications real entities at all? In this particular passage, Kendell and Jablensky seem simply to assume a radical negative view: that diagnostic categories are *simply* concepts. The suggestion seems to be that by being mere concepts, categories do not answer to the world. And that claim would also need justification. (Names for chemical elements expressed in different languages can still express the same concepts, but just because the concepts of chemistry are, tautologically, *concepts* does not undermine their claim to represent genuine features of the chemical world.) In fact, they offer a further criterion for the validity of diseases, which is mentioned the second half of the paragraph just quoted:

> Even though the authors of contemporary nomenclatures may be careful to point out that 'there is no assumption that each category of mental disorder is a completely discrete entity with absolute boundaries dividing it from other mental disorders or from no mental disorder' (DSM-IV: xxii), the mere fact that a diagnostic concept is listed in an official nomenclature and provided with a precise, complex definition tends to encourage this insidious reification. (Kendell and Jablensky 2003: 5)

The criterion for the validity of putative psychiatric syndromes is the existence of natural boundaries between them. According to Kendell and Jablensky, the 'insidious reification' occurs *despite* the fact that there may be no natural boundaries. So natural boundaries would permit a non-insidious reification:

> The crucial issue is whether psychiatric syndromes are separated from one another, and from normality, by zones of rarity or whether they are merely arbitrary loci in a multidimensional space in which variation in both symptoms and aetiology is more or less continuous. (Kendell and Jablensky 2003: 7)

The existence of boundaries between putative syndromes is, however, only one possible test of the validity of a classification. An alternative test that Kendell and Jablensky consider and reject is the development of a causal explanation, or aetiology of a syndrome. Their reasons for rejecting this alternative are as follows:

> There are several reasons why the crucial issue in determining validity is not understanding of aetiology but rather the existence of clear boundaries or qualitative differences at the level of the defining characteristic. First, understanding of aetiology is not an all-or-none issue. It often emerges in stages as a complex network of interacting events is elucidated. Second, a clear boundary may be apparent, or be demonstrated, long before the underlying aetiology is known. The histology of Creutzfeldt–Jacob disease and the other spongiform encephalopathies was recognized to be different from that of other brain diseases before abnormal prions were even conceived. The atheromatous plaques in the walls of coronary arteries, which are the defining characteristic of ischemic heart disease, were recognized as a distinct pathology, albeit one that often long preceded the onset of symptoms, several decades before their aetiology was at all well understood. It is now apparent that the aetiology of plaque formation is extremely complex, both genetically and environmentally. (Kendell and Jablensky 2003: 8)

This clear—although contestable argument—is, however, in some tension with another, earlier passage in the same paper in which underlying biological mechanism is granted some significance as a test for validity:

> Kraepelin—a staunch 'disease realist'—long believed that dementia praecox and manic-depressive insanity, defined by painstaking clinical observation of their symptoms and

outcome, represented distinct species of brain disease whose causal mechanisms would ultimately be discovered by neuropathology, experimental psychology, and genetics. Eventually, however, he abandoned his assumption that these two disorders were discrete entities and proposed instead a model that was essentially dimensional. About the same time, Jaspers wrote that 'the idea of the disease-entity is in truth an idea in Kant's sense of the word: the concept of an objective which one cannot reach … but all the same it indicates the path for fruitful research and supplies a *valid* point of orientation for particular empirical investigations'. He then added that, although 'the idea of disease-entities has become a fruitful orientation for the investigations of special psychiatry … no actual disease-entities exist'.

The relevance of this view to the present taxonomic debate in psychiatry is twofold. First, discrete disease-entities and dimensions of continuous variation are not mutually exclusive means of conceptualizing psychiatric disorders; both are compatible with a threshold model of disease and may account for different or even overlapping segments of psychiatric morbidity. Second, the surface phenomena of psychiatric illness (i.e. the clustering of symptoms, signs, course, and outcome) provide no secure basis for deciding whether a diagnostic class or rubric is valid, in the sense of delineating a specific, necessary, and sufficient biological mechanism. (Kendell and Jablensky 2003: 6, italics added)

There is thus some ambiguity in Kendell and Jablensky's precise views about the relative merits of and relationship between the existence of natural boundaries and the development of aetiological theory for establishing the validity of the classification of psychiatric syndromes. The ambiguity, however, highlights the fact that both of these competing intuitions seem reasonable marks of, or partial tests for, validity.

The same sorts of concern with correctly describing the real world have also been at the heart of a debate in the philosophy of science, which more directly concerns sciences whose understanding of causal mechanisms is more advanced than psychiatry. Again, whilst there is obviously something correct about the idea of getting the world right, it is difficult to articulate exactly what this amounts to.

Before turning to that, I will outline a second source of complexity in assessing the validity of psychiatric classification.

## The World Psychiatric Association and the idea of comprehensive diagnosis

A recent development within the World Psychiatric Association is the advocacy of a 'comprehensive' model of diagnosis. A WPA workgroup charged with formulating 'International Guidelines for Diagnostic Assessment' (IGDA) has published a guideline called 'Idiographic (personalised) Diagnostic Formulation', which recommends an idiographic component within psychiatric diagnoses. This has been put forward within the context of the development of a model of 'comprehensive diagnosis', which is described by Juan Mezzich, President of the WPA, as follows:

> The emerging comprehensive diagnostic model aims at understanding and formulating what is important in the mind, the body and the context of the person who presents for care. This is attempted by addressing the various aspects of ill- and positive- health, by interactively engaging clinicians, patient and family, and by employing categorical, dimensional *and narrative* descriptive approaches in multilevel schemas. (Mezzich 2005: 91, italics added)

Writing in the journal *Psychopathology*, the psychiatrist James Phillips describes a narrative and idiographic addition to conventional criteria-based diagnosis in this way:

> In the most simple terms, a narrative or idiographic formulation is an individual account with first-person and third-person aspects. That is, the patient tells her/his story, with its admixture of personal memories, events and symptoms, and the story is retold by the clinician. The latter's account may contain formal diagnostic, ICD-10/DSM-IV aspects, as well as psychodynamic and cultural dimensions not found in the manuals. The clinician's account may restructure the patient's presentation, emphasizing what the patient didn't emphasize and de-emphasising what the patient felt to be important. It will almost certainly contextualise the presenting symptoms into the patient's narrative, a task which the patient may not have initiated on her own. Finally, the clinician will make a judgment (or be unable to make sure a judgment) regarding the priority of the biological or the psychological in this particular presentation, and will structure the formulation accordingly ... (Phillips 2005: 182)

As mentioned in Chapter 3, the term 'idiographic' was introduced by the 19th century German philosopher Wilhelm Windelband in a debate about the methods of the human and the natural sciences. It stands in opposition to explanation based on natural laws (nomothetic) and refers instead to an individual case-based understanding:

> So we may say that the empirical sciences seek in the knowledge of reality either the general in the form of the natural law or the particular in the historically determined form [Gestalt]. They consider in one part the ever enduring form, in the other part the unique content, determined within itself, of an actual happening. The one comprises sciences of law, the other sciences of events; the former teaches what always is, the latter what once was. If one may resort to neologisms, it can be said that scientific thought is in the one case nomothetic, in the other idiographic. (Windelband (1894) 1998: 13)

What kind of intelligibility might be essentially individualistic and based on a 'case of one'? The most natural way to understand 'idiographic' is as a meaning-based variety of understanding, belonging to the 'space of reasons', rather than the 'realm of law' (McDowell 1994). This also fits Windelband's reference to history as a suitable example.

This, however, introduces some complexity to the matter. Just how individualist is reason-based understanding? (Recall that in this context idiographic understanding is introduced in contrast to the criterial understanding of DSM and ICD models of diagnosis.) Two models mentioned in Chapter 2 may be helpful. *Simulation theory* in the philosophy of mind and *particularism* about moral judgement.

In the debate about knowledge of other minds, simulation theory opposes theory theory by denying that one needs to have knowledge of a theory of mind to form judgements about other people's mental states. One needs, instead, merely to have a mind and to be able imaginatively to put oneself into the predicament of another and, thus, determine what one would think in those circumstances, weighing opposing factors or reasons. Such judgements are made without the requirement of a general theory of reasons.

In the debate about moral judgement, particularism opposes principlism in denying that successful moral judgement can be encoded in a set of principles. Instead, it turns on careful scrutiny of the moral features, the moral reasons that make up particular cases and that pull in opposing directions. Again, such judgements are made without the requirement of a general theory of moral reasons.

So, in the case at hand, a narrative or idiographic formulation is not derived from a theory of human nature or a general theory of reasons, but is instead the result of careful attention to the accounts, narratives and behaviour of subjects. That negative characterisation contrasts with conventional DSM- or ICD-based nomothetic, criterial diagnosis. On the other hand, however, there is a principled limit to the extent to which such a formulation can be individualistic. This other limit is avoidance of what has been called the 'Myth of the Given' by the US philosopher Wilfrid Sellars (1912–1989), who uses it to characterise a form of foundationalism based on experiences that ground, but do not themselves depend on, other conceptualised beliefs:

> One of the forms taken by the Myth of the Given is the idea that there is, indeed *must be*, a structure of particular matter of fact such that (a) each fact can not only be noninferentially known to be the case, but presupposes no other knowledge either of particular matter of fact, or of general truths; and (b) such that the noninferential knowledge of facts belonging to this structure constitutes the ultimate court of appeals for all factual claims—particular and general—about the world. It is important to note that I characterized the knowledge of fact belonging to this stratum as not only noninferential, but as presupposing no knowledge of other matter of fact, whether particular or general. (Sellars 1997: 68–9)

The Myth of the Given is a form of epistemological foundationalism which, for reasons beyond the scope of this book, Sellars convincingly undermines (see also McDowell 1994; Thornton 2004: 209–24). The most basic epistemological level always presupposes conceptual connections to other states. Thus, in virtue of those conceptual connections, no narrative account of an individual subject is fully idiographic. The application of concepts—within a narrative—are essentially 'one to many' relations. In fact, Phillips also recognises limits to the extent to which an individualistic formulation really is idiographic:

> Narrative, idiographic formulations approach the question of generalization differently from most medical diagnoses. In one sense, the notion of an idiographic diagnosis is an oxymoron; the idiographic account is an individual account and thus resists any diagnostic categorization of the patient. On the other hand, we do use narrative generalizations; they are just not the categorical, criterial structures of ICD-10/DSM-IV. (Phillips 2005: 182–3)

This suggests a kind of practical balance. As far as is possible, a narrative formulation is individualistic in that it aims to capture the details of individual subjects and it eschews theories of human nature. At the same time, however, it does this using a rational structure of meaning-based concepts and, thus, deploys an essential generality.

If psychiatric diagnosis is to include a narrative-based and, as far is possible, idiographic ingredient, if the basic classificatory judgement of psychiatry is to include this element, then what of its validity? Note, first, the contrast with classification in chemistry. There, the validity of the Periodic Table is displayed in classificatory judgements, which are essentially general. Samples are described as instances of general types, which possess a great deal of systematic import, in Hempel's phrase. Validity in chemistry is underpinned by the use of *general* kinds.

The WPA's suggestion pulls in the other direction: narrative components in a comprehensive diagnosis are tailored to individual cases in a way which seems, by definition, to undermine systematic import, in Hempel's phrase. Does this undermine the validity of classifications based on this approach? The difficulty in answering the question is that assessing validity seems to require stepping outside one's beliefs to measure them against the world, to check that they line up, but that, of course, is impossible. So it seems that one needs a less direct measure of validity. To help address this need I will now turn to some lessons from the philosophy of science.

## 3. Lessons from the philosophy of science

In the early part of the 20th century, many philosophers of science advocated an instrumentalist and positivistic attitude towards science. They argued that theoretical claims about the world did not function as literally descriptive claims.

In part, this emphasis was the result of the precise way in which observation was credited with a central role in science. The Logical Empiricists attempted to defend the central role of impartial observation by distinguishing between an independent language of observational concepts and a dependent language of theoretical concepts. Given this distinction, it was plausible (although by no means mandatory) to construe statements framed with observational concepts as making genuine empirical claims, whilst construing theoretical statements as merely playing a heuristic role in organising the former. When so construed, theoretical statements are not themselves fact stating, or capable of truth and falsity. They play a role that is not one of assertion, but rather as an instrument for organising genuinely fact-stating claims. In other words, theoretical statements do not possess any kind of validity. They are not aimed at getting things right.

Such a view reflects a positivistic attitude to the connection between meaningfulness and verification. Since theoretical statements cannot themselves be directly verified and, instead, receive whatever confirmation or refutation indirectly via observational statements, they are regarded by many as possessing a different kind of meaning from verifiable observational statements.

Whilst this attitude is still found amongst philosophically-influenced practising scientists, it is rare amongst philosophers of science. One reason for this is the attack on the distinction between theory and observation that threatens a firm semantic distinction between the meaning of observation statements and that of theoretical statements. If theoretical and observational statements are made in the same language—if no separation is possible between theoretical and observational concepts—then theoretical statements cannot be sharply marked out as playing a different kind of role. The difference between theory and observation is a matter of degree (see Fulford *et al.* 2006: 288–315).

In place of a positivistic and instrumentalist view of scientific theory, the current orthodoxy is a form of realism about science called Scientific Realism. 'Realism', however, describes more than one philosophical position. It is, in the philosopher J. L. Austin's (1911–60) phrase, a 'trouser word':

> Next, 'real' is what we may call a trouser-word. It is usually thought, and I dare say usually rightly thought, that what one might call the affirmative use of a term is basic—that, to understand 'x,' we need to know what it is to be x, or to be an x, and that knowing this apprises us of what it is not to be x, not to be an x. But with 'real' (as we briefly noted earlier) it is the negative use that wears the trousers. (Austin 1962: 70)

For this reason, it is clearest to understand realism by looking at what it is contrasted with. In recent philosophy of science, the most influential critique of realism has been offered by Bas Van Fraassen in the form of the articulation of Constructive Empiricism. As I will explain, it shares some of the features of a positivistic view, but also shares some of the underlying metaphysical assumptions of scientific realism. Responses to Constructive Empiricism will suggest ways of underpinning validity, but in ways that will not help comprehensive diagnosis for which a different approach will be required.

## Constructive Empiricism

Outlined in his book *The Scientific Image*, Van Fraassen's position is a form of anti-realism, but it is important to be clear just what it is that he denies. One element of a *realist* attitude to science is that science aims to give us a 'literally true story of what the world is like', but this claim itself involves two aspects:

> the language is to be literally construed; and so construed, the account is true. This divides the anti-realists into two sorts. The first sort holds that science is or aims to be true, properly (but not literally) construed. The second holds that that the language of science should be literally construed, but its theories need not be true to be good. The anti-realism I shall advocate belongs to the second sort. (Van Fraassen 1999: 187)

Van Fraassen's position is thus *not* the same as a positivistic or instrumentalist account. Those accounts deny that theoretical statements are capable of truth or falsity, but serve a different, purely organisational, role. In other words, they can be 'true' in so far as they organise successfully, but this is not the same as literal truth. By contrast, Van Fraassen accepts the realist view that theoretical scientific statements are either true or false when construed literally. Just as they appear to do, theoretical statements really do make claims about the world. This marks out a *semantic* realist position. Furthermore, Van Fraassen takes a further *metaphysical* view about the nature of truth. Theoretical statements are true (or false), in virtue of how the world is or what the facts are. Truth is a matter of correspondence with a mind-independent objective world. This is a form of metaphysical realism.

However, Van Fraassen combines these views with a form of *epistemological* anti-realism. Although theoretical statements are construed as (really) either true or false in virtue of the world, we can never arrive at sufficient evidence to *discover* or to *know*, which statements are true and which are false. Thus, we should refrain from committing ourselves to the truth of theoretical statements—to do so is to take an unnecessary risk. Instead, science should aim merely to arrive at theories that are empirically adequate. Acceptance of a theory should similarly involve merely belief that it is empirically adequate. A theory is empirically adequate if and only if 'what it says about the observable things and events in this world is true—exactly if it saves the phenomena'. We should aim at nothing beyond this. Applied to psychiatric taxonomy this amounts to the claim that the aim of validity should be restricted to observational matters and not to theoretical or aetiological accounts.

So characterised, Constructive Empiricism is prescriptive. It says that one *should not* accept the truth of theoretical statements. But this prescription is not arbitrary and results from epistemological arguments about what can and cannot be known. In *The Scientific Image*, Van Fraassen's argument for Constructive Empiricism takes the form of a series of attacks on epistemological realism. In effect, he argues that, since believing in the truth or theories involves more than merely in their empirical adequacy, there should be an argument for this extra step and that no such argument is successful. This may seem an unusual way of apportioning the burden of proof. Since Constructive Empiricism is counter-intuitive, an argument might be needed to motivate it. One such argument might run as follows:

- At any given time, the only evidence for a theory is the set of relevant observations already made.

- For any finite body of observations, there is always more than one theory which is consistent with it. These different theories differ in what they say about unobservables. (They might also differ in what they say about future observables, but I will ignore this point for the moment.)

- Since the only evidence for theories concerns the observable realm, there is no way of deciding which theory correctly describes the unobservable realm.

- Thus, we should not take the risk of choosing between these different theories and accept instead what they all have in common: their descriptions of the observable realm. We should, in other words, adopt Constructive Empiricism.

- However, since all the consequences which can matter for us are observable we also lose nothing by this.

This argument is not watertight, but the basic assumption that drives it—and that will not be questioned in what follows—is the thesis of the Underdetermination of Theory by Data, often associated with the American pragmatist philosopher W. V. O. Quine (1908–2000).

There are stronger and weaker versions of this thesis. At its strongest, it claims that even given all the possible evidence that we could amass, there would remain more than one theory consistent with it. Some care has to be taken in how one construes 'all possible evidence'. If it means simply 'all the facts', then it is hard to see how this would not determine which theory were true. Instead, it has to be construed—even in this strong version of the thesis—as meaning 'all the evidence that it is possible for we humans, having extended our senses through instruments, to amass'. There is, however, a weaker thesis that will serve our present purposes. It is the claim that for any finite body of evidence, there is always more than one theory consistent with it.

Even this weak reading of the Underdetermination Thesis appears to justify Van Fraassen's claim. Theories that are consistent with the data will have to differ one from another in what they say either about future observable matters or about unobservable matters. A version of Constructive Empiricism that restricted our beliefs to past observable states of affairs would be one that followed Hume's sceptical attack on induction (see Chapter 6). This would be a radical position that denied that we could know anything about the future. Van Fraassen's position is more reasonable. Granting that induction is some-times possible, he concentrates instead on those aspects of theories that concern unobservable matters and says that we should withhold judgment on these. The reason for this restriction is the claim that the only rational method of judging between theories is evidence and that, by definition, there cannot be evidence which concerns the unobservable realm. That would require that the realm were not unobservable after all.

Coupled with the claim that we cannot have knowledge of the unobservable realm, Van Fraassen also suggests that we lose nothing by abstaining from judgment about it. All that can interest us are the observable consequences of theories, because these are the only aspects that have practical consequences. Thus, we should not take the risk of commitment to particular accounts of unobservables, but neither is this of any practical loss.

We can now see the difference between Van Fraassen's view of unobservables in general and Thomas Szasz' view of mental illness described in Chapter 1. Szasz argues that there are no such things as mental illnesses, at least as we have previously thought of them. He denies that any such notion is coherent. Van Fraassen does not deny that there are unobservables. Furthermore, he thinks that claims about them are as true or false as claims about chairs and tables, and true in the same literal way. However, he thinks that we cannot *know* which are true and which false. The difference between Van Fraassen and Szasz is akin to that between agnosticism and atheism. (Although this analogy is complicated by the fact that Szasz does not deny the existence of mental illness *as* societal constructs or life problems.)

Van Fraassen's position may capture the intuitions of Kendell and Jablensky in the passage quoted earlier when they say that 'Thoughtful clinicians have long been aware that diagnostic categories are simply concepts, justified only by whether they provide a useful framework for organizing and explaining the complexity of clinical experience in order to derive inferences about outcome and to guide decisions about treatment.' Perhaps they mean that thoughtful clinicians should believe merely in the empirical adequacy of diagnostic cate-gories and their observable consequences through treatment guidance. If so, this raises the question of whether there is, after all, reason to believe more, to believe that diagnostic categories actually are valid.

## Inference to the best explanation

The Underdetermination Thesis played a key role in the brief sketch of an argument above. That thesis is based on the claim that there is more than one theory that is *consistent* with any finite body of evidence. That claim is remarkably weak, however. It simply means that there is more than one theory that is not incompatible with the data, whose falsity is not implied by it. Thus, the claim that there is more than one such theory may come as no surprise.

In general, however, we think that there is a stronger relation between data and theory than mere consistency. We think of data as *supporting* theory. It can provide positive evidence or warrant for our beliefs. That is what is involved in taking events in the past as a *reason* for holding beliefs about what will happen in the future. Inductive inference involves not just eliminating theories that are inconsistent with past events, but also using past events as a guide to choosing between the consistent theories that remain. The fact that Van Fraassen accepts that this is possible is shown by his acceptance of theories that make predictions about future observable matters. This leaves the problem that in the case of unobservables we cannot begin to establish inductive generalisations linking the macro- and microscopic because we are never in a position to check the microscopic.

As the US philosopher of science Richard Boyd points out, there is another kind of relation between theory and data provided by *explanation*. If a theory enjoys explanatory success, then, according to Boyd, it is likely to be true, or likely to be largely or approximately true. This suggests that there is a way of supporting detailed claims about unobservable realms. One looks for the best explanation of observable phenomena whether or not it employs unobservable or microscopic features:

> The proposal that scientific realism might be required in order to adequately explain the instrumental reliability of scientific methodology can be motivated by re-examining the principal constructivist argument against scientific realism. The constructivist asks, 'What must the world be like in order that a methodology so theory-dependent as ours could constitute a way of finding out what's true?' She answers: 'The world would have to be largely defined or constituted by the theoretical tradition which defines that methodology'. It is clear that another answer is at least possible: the world might be one in which the laws and theories embodied in our actual theoretical tradition are approximately true. In that case, the methodology of science might progress dialectically. Our methodology, based on approximately true theories, would be a reliable guide to the discovery of new results and the improvement of older theories ... I argue that the reliability of theory-dependent judgements of projectibility and degrees of confirmation can only be satisfactorily explained on the assumption that the theoretical claims embodied in the background theories which determine those judgements are relevantly approximately true ... (Boyd 1999: 207)

Another realist philosopher, Ernan McMullin, gives the example of Galileo's explanation of the changing shadows on the moon which invokes lunar mountains (McMullin 1987). Because lunar mountains are the best explanation of the shadows, there is good reason, given the existence of the shadows, to believe in the existence of lunar mountains. In fact, this example would be classed by Van Fraassen as concerning observables since lunar mountains could eventually be observed with the naked eye, but the same kind of explanation-based strategy could also be applied in microscopic cases.

In the case of Galileo and lunar mountains, the qualification 'best' in 'inference to the best explanation' may seem superfluous. What other explanation of the shadows could there be? However, given the status of the astronomical telescope as a scientific instrument at the time, even in this case an alternative might have been to explain the observed phenomenon away as a mere artefact of the instrument. Mere 'noise' is often an appropriate rival explanation in the case of putative observations made with complex modern instruments (whether space telescopes, vats of cleaning fluid for the detection of neutrinos, humble electron microscopes, or EEG machines). In the case of lunar shadows, that rival explanation becomes less compelling once the varied phenomena can be repeatedly observed, changing in accordance with the relative position of the sun. So, in the case of competing explanations, one should look for the best explanation and infer the truth of its explanans, but an explanation may still be the best explanation even if it is the only (plausible) one.

Scientific Realism is typically regarded as the combination of semantic, metaphysical and epistemological views. Van Fraassen holds realist views about both the semantics and the metaphysics of science. Scientific statements, literally construed, are either true or false, and they are true or false in virtue of the state of a mind-independent world, but a realist like Boyd or McMullin disagrees with Van Fraassen's epistemological anti-realism by claiming that we can also claim to know the truth or approximate truth of the full range of scientific statements.

How might this argument apply to the validity, or otherwise, of psychiatric taxonomy? The key test is whether the taxonomy furnishes the materials for good explanations of observable phenomena. So, on a plausible view that such explanation is likely to be causal, Boyd and McMullin support the view that Kendell and Jablensky reject in favour of the existence of natural boundaries between categories. The test for validity of diagnosis is the development of aetiological theory thus pulling against Hempel's interim advocacy of more observational terms (and in favour of his further praise of systematic import).

Despite the widespread defence of inference to the best explanation, the issue of whether explanatory success can ground claims about the truth of scientific claims across the board is also contested—in a different way from Van Fraassen—by the contemporary American philosopher of science and of physics, Nancy Cartwright.

## Cartwright's inference to the most probable cause

Roughly speaking, Cartwright is a realist about those unobservable entities that are invoked to explain observable effects. She rejects inference to the best (theoretical) explanation, but accepts inference to 'the most probable cause'. There are two general arguments that underpin this distinction.

- A general scepticism about theoretical explanation. Theoretical explanation, she argues, is a matter of providing a unifying account of diverse phenomena. In the physical sciences, this is provided by mathematical theories from which statements about observable phenomena can be derived, but such theoretical explanations do not presuppose the truth of the explanatory theory. That a description of an observable phenomenon can be derived from a theory coupled with the fact that the description is true does not imply that the theory is also true. (I will return briefly to this claim below.)

- An empirical claim about scientific theories. Cartwright argues that there is often more than one incompatible, theoretical account that could, in principle, be applied to the same phenomena. As a matter of fact, scientists take a pragmatic attitude to choosing which theoretical treatment to use depending on which is most appropriate to any particular case. Appropriateness, in this case, depends on ease of mathematical application, as well as accuracy, but if the theories used in explanation had to be true, then no such pragmatic attitude would be possible.

Cartwright thus differs from Van Fraassen in distinguishing theoretical explanations from causal explanations. The key difference between the two cases is that higher level theories do not *bring about* the lower level descriptions which can be derived from them, whereas causes do bring about their effects. Thus, if a causal explanation were to fail to pick out real entities, it would fail as an explanation. By contrast, if a high level theoretical explanation turns out to be false, it might still organise the lower level descriptions of the world in an efficient and clear manner.

This contrast can be brought out with an example from psycho analysis. Consider as the range of observable phenomena to be explained the sorts of apparently unintentional actions and slips of the tongue, which Freud describes (especially in *The Psychopathology of Everyday Life* (Freud 2002)). Now consider two sorts of explanation of these. One cites the truth of Freud's complex system of sub-personal mental agents whose characteristic interaction is precisely described in Freudian meta psychological theory. The other simply cites the existence of such agents as id, ego, superego as the causes of the phenomena. Cartwright suggests that if the evidence for both accounts were broadly favourable we should, nevertheless, not believe in the truth of Freud's overall higher level theory, but we should, in the absence of better rival accounts, believe in the existence of the entities he postulates. This is further reinforced if one can manipulate such entities, through, in this case, analysis.

Of course, from our perspective, belief in neither may seem very attractive, but this helps reiterate an implicit point that all these argument forms are, from a logical point of view, invalid. True premises can lead to false conclusions. Furthermore, justification is context dependent. At the turn of the last century, belief in such mental entities or agents may well have been justified given the evidence available even if it would no longer be.

The argument so far summarised, however, is open to the objection that Cartwright is wrong to claim that theoretical explanation does not require the truth of the higher level theories. Surely, runs the objection, if a theory is false it cannot be an explanation of anything. (Similarly, if a belief is false it cannot form the basis of knowledge. There is no 'false knowledge'. Similarly, there are no 'false explanations'.) However, Cartwright has a broader thesis to provide indirect support for her claims about the nature of theoretical explanation. She claims that it is no coincidence that high level laws are all false.

The argument for this startling claim is contained in her book punningly titled *How the Laws of Physics Lie* (Cartwright 1983). The main idea is that explanation and truth are incompatible goals. To be explanatory, a theory must abstract from the descriptions of individual cases an underlying pattern. An example is Newton's law of gravitational attraction, which states that the force exerted on any particle in the universe by any other is proportional to the product of their masses divided by the square of their distance apart. However, such a theory neglects other forces, which also act on particles, such as electromagnetic forces. To be accurate one would have to say 'all other things being equal', or *ceteris paribus*, 'the force is proportional to …'. Since other things are rarely equal, such a law, although true, would not be explanatory. In general the higher level the theory or law, the more explanatory, but the less true.

Again there is a natural counter-argument. One might say that the law of gravitational attraction gives the force *due to gravity* and that the resultant force acting on a particle depends on the vector sum of this force and all other forces. Aside from some specific arguments against the reality of the component forces involved in that calculation, Cartwright's general argument is that, for laws with *ceteris paribus* clauses, there is no general analogue of vector addition. For example, Snell's law, which governs refraction, applies only to isotropic media and so should be read as relying on a *ceteris paribus* clause. If other things are not equal, if the media are not isotropic, there is no mechanical way of producing an appropriate refinement. In general, there is no neutral way of combining the effects of different *ceteris paribus* laws, which all apply to some specific circumstance. Outside basic sciences, however, most laws rely on 'all other things being equal' clauses.

This view is a reflection of a more fundamental and dramatic view of nature:

> I imagine that natural objects are much like people in societies. Their behaviour is constrained by some specific laws and by a handful of general principles, but it is not determined in detail even statistically. What happens on most occasions is dictated by no law at all. This is not a metaphysical picture that I urge. My claim is that this picture is as plausible as the alternative. God may have written just a few laws and grown tired. (Cartwright 1983: 49)

> The laws that describe this world are a patchwork, not a pyramid. They do not take after the simple, elegant and abstract structure of a system of axioms and theorems. Rather they look like—and steadfastly stick to looking like—science as we know it: apportioned into disciplines, apparently arbitrarily grown up; governing different sets of properties at different levels of abstraction; pockets of great precision; large parcels of qualitative maxims resisting precise formulation; erratic overlaps; here and there, once in a while, corners that line up, but mostly ragged edges; and always the cover of law just loosely attached to the jumbled world of material things. For all we know, most of what happens in nature occurs by hap, subject to no law at all. What happens is more like an outcome of negotiation between domains than the logical conse-quence of a system of order. (Cartwright 1999: 1)

This basic picture—which amounts to a limited form of metaphysical, as well as epistemological anti-realism—is both radical and contested. The more frequent assumption is that determining the basic micro-physical constituents of the world determines the chances of subsequent events ('determines the chances' takes account of micro-physical indeterminacy). This latter assump-tion is sometimes called the 'completeness of physics', taken to mean the potential completeness of physics, or of a future physics. It plays a role, also, in reductionist accounts of higher level sciences to basic sciences, but although it is a widely held view, the completeness of physics is not analytically true. Nor is it knowable *a priori*. Cartwright points out that an alternative is also possible and, furthermore, that existing evidence seems—to her at least—to point against it.

Before I assess in a little more detail the implications of both the inference to the best explanation and the inference to the most probable cause for psychiatric taxonomy, I will outline a different kind of response to both real-ism and anti-realism in the philosophy of science that calls into question the possibility of assessing validity.

## The natural ontological attitude: from what perspective can we assess scientific validity?

The discussion of philosophy of science so far has focused on the epistemological claim that we can come to know about hidden aspects of the world via science. But it is worth remembering that this claim is made against a background of metaphysical realism. It is to that that I will now turn by considering Arthur Fine's 'natural ontological attitude' (1986). He also provides a clue to the resolution of the epistemological debate that will also shed light on the comments by Kendell and Jablensky.

Fine begins by arguing against the effectiveness of realism as an account of the success of science. The epistemological anti-realist is characterised by Fine as resisting the claim that a successful explanation is likely to be true. This fits Van Fraassen and Cartwright (and others). Realists claim, by contrast, that realism is the only account that does not make the success of science a miracle, but the argument used to support epistemological realism is thus of the following form:

◆ Scientific realism explains the success of science and, thus, it (scientific realism) is likely to be true.

In other words, it trades on just the inference from explanatory success to truth that epistemological anti-realists deny. Fine's key claim is that deploying realism to explain the success of science simply reiterates the form of reasoning that is in question.

It is worth taking this point slowly. The challenge that scientific realism takes on is to justify belief in the reality of those individuals, properties, relations, processes and so forth, used in well-supported explanatory hypotheses. In the case at hand—psychiatric taxonomy—the challenge is to justify belief that the categories set out in DSM and ICD diagnostic manuals really do answer to genuine structural features of our mental lives and mental health, and ill health.

In this context, realism is itself a high level hypothesis that, realists argue, is supported by the data. It is the hypothesis that accepted scientific theories are, indeed, approximately true, rather than merely empirically adequate, where 'being approximately true' is taken to denote an extra-theoretical relation between theories and the world. Thus, to address doubts over the reality of relations posited by everyday scientific hypotheses, the realist introduces realism as, itself, a further high level explanatory hypothesis, which posits just such a relation (approximate truth). Surely, Fine argues, anyone serious about the issue of realism and with an open mind about it, would be behaving inconsistently if he or she were to accept the realist move as satisfactory. Just because realism 'best explains' scientific practice need not indicate that it is true.

Although Fine argues against traditional epistemological realism, he does not support a form of epistemological anti-realism either. Instead, he argues that the debate is itself the result of a mistaken metaphysical urge. What both realists and anti-realists should—and he claims typically do—accept is a 'homely line'. This core position comprises an acceptance of well-grounded scientific claims as having the same status as everyday knowledge claims, but they go on to qualify this common core with further metaphysical claims.

Before going on to summarise those metaphysical additions, it is worth emphasising that Fine's homely line would not be acceptable to Van Fraassen. He, by contrast, distinguishes between claims that would be regarded as of equal status by Fine because his distinction between claims made about observables and unobservables is revisionary of ordinary scientific practice. Things are less clear with regard to Cartwright. There is some reason to believe that Cartwright's distrust of high level scientific theories is, itself, an accurate reflection of scientific practice. This is certainly one of the arguments she presents for it. Scientists are, she suggests, pragmatically open to the use of any of a range of different and incompatible theories, selecting one on the basis of its usefulness. On the other hand, a sharp distinction between realism about theories and entities would be revisionary in that a well-established theory might well be accepted as having the same status as the claim that electrons exist.

Fine, then, suggests that realists and anti-realists add to the basic core position a further philosophical gloss. Anti-realists provide a reinterpretation of truth. This might be an idealist claim that nothing can exist independently of human experience. It might be the claim that the truth of a belief consists in its coherence with other beliefs or it might be the claim that truth just is being useful as some pragmatists claim. Each of these modifications re-interprets the common core. (Recall, however, that Van Fraassen suggested that there were two forms of anti-realism. The first sort rejects the idea that scientific statements could be true. The second holds that that the language of science should be literally construed, but its theories need not be too true to be good. On Fine's account, anti-realism is of the former kind. Van Fraassen claimed that his Constructive Empiricism was of the latter.)

Fine's characterisation of what a realist adds to the common core is simpler: 'what the realist adds on is a desk-thumping, foot-stamping shout of "Really!"'. The reason for this is that:

> The realist, as it were, tries to stand outside the arena watching the ongoing game [of science] and then tries to judge (from this external point of view) what the point is. It is, he says, about some area external to the game. The realist, I think, is fooling himself. For he cannot (really!) stand outside the arena, nor can he survey some area off the playing field and mark it out as what the game is about.' (Fine 1986: 131)

Fine's point here reflects a basic worry throughout this chapter. How can a worry or a corresponding reassurance about the validity of psychiatric taxonomy be expressed? How can the question of whether it cuts nature at its joints even be explained?

Having suggested that both realism and anti-realism attempt to add something to a common homely line, but that this is a philosophically questionable aim, Fine suggests that the best philosophical response is to adopt the homely line by itself without adding anything to it. One should adopt merely a 'natural ontological attitude', which is faithful to the beliefs and commitments of practising science. Thus, the only guide to what is real are the methods that are internal to scientific work. Philosophy cannot bring a fruitful external perspective to this issue. This is not to deny that philosophical reflection has any bearing on what is real, but such reflection should be a proper part of scientific method and not an attempt at an Archimedean perspective from outside science.

Fine's account is attractive because of its simultaneous distancing from both realism and anti-realism, and because of its emphasis on a naturalistic solution. The degree of realism one should adopt to a subject matter should depend on the local scientific case for it, but it is also clear that Fine is characterising a different kind of debate from the one with which this section began. The natural ontological attitude is distinguished from realism and the latter is characterised as trying to say something further, something illicit. However, in the discussion of Constructive Empiricism above, belief in specific claims about unobservables—which comprises a rejection of that form of epistemic anti-realism and would often be part of a natural ontological attitude—was called realism. Fine's description of realism appears to be not merely an opposition to a specific epistemological anti-realist attack on some class of beliefs— unobservables, high level theories—but a further claim. It is an attempt to step outside our practices and provide them with further philosophical foundations.

This point can be spelt out like this. Boyd and McMullin argue (as described above) that the best explanation of the success of science was that its theories (about unobservables) were approximately true and that this suggested that those theories were, indeed, approximately true. If this argument is construed as a piece of scientific reasoning—perhaps a standard piece of arguing from effects to inferred causes to block Van Fraassen's worry—it surely lies *within* the natural ontological attitude and does not amount to a further tendentious form of realism.

If, on the other hand, this argument is adopted as an attempt to provide additional reassurance that the claims which science makes as true really are true, then it does amount to a further gratuitous form of realism and Fine's argument against it is well directed. What would be the point of this further claim? Against what position could it be directed? The most obvious answer is that it could be used against a metaphysical anti-realist: someone who denied that we could begin to describe a world independent of ourselves, that apparently world-involving claims are really claims about sense-data or ideas.

Thus, Fine might be seen as running together issues that are best characterised as part of an epistemological debate and issues from a metaphysical debate. However, his solution to both is a form of philosophical quietism. To determine those elements of a science in which one should believe, one should turn to the science itself. One should reject philosophical prescriptions about which beliefs are sound and which not. That is a local matter, but one should refrain from attempts to provide extra-scientific foundations for such reasoning by saying, for example, that science as a whole must be right because it is successful. That amounts merely to a table-thumping cry of 'really!' and adds nothing to the debate.

## The application of lessons from philosophy of science to psychiatric classification

So far, this section of the chapter has outlined the kind of inference that is justified within science from observable to unobservable matters. Van Fraassen argues that such inference is never justified. Boyd argues that it is whenever it is grounded in an *explanation* of observable phenomena. Cartwright argues that it is justified, but only if the explanations in question cite the *causes* of observable phenomena and not just higher level theories from which the explanandum can be derived. How do these arguments shed light on the debate about psychiatric validity?

One lesson is that there are a number of plausible tests for the validity of scientific theory. The broader explanatory framework, the appeal to causal factors and even the possibility of casually manipulating underlying factors all contribute to evidence for the claim that a taxonomy does get matters broadly right. So if psychiatric taxonomy fits with explanatory and aetiological theories, especially theories that identify means of intervening, that is a good sign of their validity.

However, another conclusion, following from Fine's analysis, is that such bootstrapping is limited. Fine suggests that if realist arguments are construed as attempts to validate—or undermine—scientific reasoning from a perspective outside science, then, although they highlight some of the difficulties of scientific reasoning, they cannot succeed in legislating for good scientific practice. This is because it is impossible to take the sort of external perspective on science that these arguments seem to require. All the virtues of taxonomy mentioned above are merely virtues seen from within the perspective of a particular approach to scientific psychiatry, not a comment on that somehow from the outside.

What then should we make of Kendell and Jablensky's claim that clinicians should think of diagnostic categories as 'simply concepts, justified only by whether they provide a useful framework for organizing and explaining the complexity of clinical experience in order to derive inferences about outcome and to guide decisions about treatment'? It depends what precise claim they are making.

They may be advocating something like Van Fraassen's Constructive Empiricism: a form of agnosticism about whether psychiatric classification really is valid, but if so, the success of the classification in guiding treatment, in successfully intervening in subjects' health, might provide an argument for supposing the classification to be valid. That would be to follow the advice of Cartwright in emphasising practical manipulation of unobservable entities—in this case disease-entities.

On the other hand, they may be saying something stronger: that classifications could not possibly be anything more than 'mere concepts', constructs that are neither true nor false, and merely help organise data. That would be a form of instrumentalism. If so, then Fine's diagnosis suggests that it is an ill-founded attempt to step outside the natural ontological attitude proper to psychiatric theory.

How does the philosophy of science debate impact on the idea of adding narrative elements to comprehensive diagnosis? Here, things are a little more complex. The tests of validity suggested by Boyd and Cartwright do not seem to apply to individualistic narrative accounts of subjects.

To begin with, Boyd's deployment of the 'inference to the best explanation' is based on the idea that a theory that best explains some observable phenomenon acquires, by that fact, justification. It is more likely to be true or valid. In other words, it is reasonable to infer to the truth of the underlying theory that best explains the phenomenon. So if this were to apply to a narrative component of a comprehensive diagnosis then that would have to be construed as a theory of underlying states that best explains behaviour. There are two difficulties with this.

First, for such an inference to apply to an account couched in the 'space of reasons', it would presuppose a particular kind of account of reasons or mental states. It would have to be one in which mental states were construed as underlying causal entities: the unobserved causes of observable behaviour. This is the view taken by 'functionalism' within the philosophy of mind, but functionalist accounts of mental states face grave difficulties in accounting for the normative and rational nature of the mind. It is this that lies at the heart of criticisms of functionalism (see, e.g. Heal 1995; McDowell 1998b), but is also underpinned by the argument from Wittgenstein described in Chapter 4 (Wittgenstein 1953; Heal 1995; McDowell 1998b: 325–340). So inference to the best explanation can only apply if one adopts a particular view of the metaphysics of mind of which there is reason to be sceptical.

Secondly, even if a functionalist account of mind were to be accepted, it would stand in sharp contrast to the aim of narrative or idiographic elements in diagnosis. The purpose of such elements in a comprehensive diagnosis is to capture individuality by contrast with the generality of criterial diagnosis in accord with DSM and ICD guidelines. That is in direct conflict with the idea of a functionalist account of the mind in which mental states are characterised by general causal connections between perceptions, mental states and behaviour. The individuality stressed by an idiographic approach prevents the application of a functionalist analysis of mind and, hence, inference to the best explanation.

The same general characteristics of an idiographic account preclude such elements of a comprehensive diagnosis passing Cartwright's test. In general, in psychiatry, success in identifying causal elements that explain psychiatric symptoms has been limited. But in the case at hand, the idea of narrative accounts does not seem to be of the right sort to reveal underlying causal agents in contrast to a higher level theory. The problem is that the test of a narrative account of a subject's life or experiences is narrative fit. Whilst there might be a sufficiently rough and ready distinction between theory and entity in the case of, say, electrons, that seems much less plausible in the case of, say, jealous resentment. In the latter case, it is much less plausible to suggest that such an entity might have causal effect on behaviour however it is described by 'narrative theory'. Entity and theory are too closely bound together for Cartwright's separation to be useful.

Does that suggest that there is no hope of narrative elements of comprehensive diagnoses possessing validity? The tests of validity that Boyd and Cartwright suggest are both expressed in nomothetic or realm of law terms. Against these tests, an individualised, idiographic or space of reasons element is bound to fail, but that is to judge such additions to psychiatric taxonomy against the wrong standard. Is there a standard by which to test the validity of a narrative account of a subject's life and experiences?

One clue comes from the fact that the test should apply not only to any individual account, but also to the very terms and concepts used to frame any such account. Think of the use of terms like 'passive aggressive' in everyday dialogue in Woody Allen films. Individual narratives are framed using concepts that carry with them particular ways of making sense of subjects and all such concepts are open to critical scrutiny.

In broad terms, narrative accounts of an individual's life have to answer both to individual circumstances and also to a broader structure of rationality. The conditions of adequacy are overall conditions of fit even if, in line with Fine's natural ontological attitude, there is no external perspective to judge that outside what makes sense to us. Adapting a suggestive passage from McDowell suggests the test in question:

> Like any thinking, [narrative] thinking is under a standing obligation to reflect about and criticise the standards by which, at any time, it takes itself to be governed ... Now it is a key point that for such reflective criticism, the appropriate image is Neurath's, in which a sailor overhauls his ship while it is afloat. This does not mean such reflection cannot be radical. One can find oneself called on to jettison parts of one's inherited ways of thinking; and, though this is harder to place in Neurath's image, weaknesses that reflection discloses in inherited ways of thinking can dictate the formation of new concepts and conceptions. But the essential thing is one can reflect only from the midst of the way of thinking one is reflecting about. (McDowell 1994: 81)

Thus, the test for the validity of narrative formulations is in the end a matter of generality: the generality of patterns of what makes rational sense. This is not a matter of algorithm or rules. It is instead a matter of judgement, but the judgements are made using concepts that have essentially general application.

## 4. **Conclusions**

Recent concern with the validity of psychiatric classification has a number of motivations. The most striking stems from the debate about anti-psychiatry discussed in Chapter 1. At the heart of that debate is the question of whether mental illness is essentially evaluative or not. If it is then this might seem to undermine its status as a valid description of the world. Indeed, this might explain Szasz' comment that his assertion that mental illness is a myth is a premiss not conclusion, so direct might seem the connection between the presence of values and a lack of validity (Szasz 2004: 321).

In fact, however, the connection is not straightforward. Even if mental illness is an essentially evaluative notion that need not rule out the validity of psychiatric classification. The argument that it must is underpinned by a neo-Humean view of values that is open to criticism: primarily that the distinction between value-free worldly features and world-free evaluative sentiments cannot be drawn. Without a neo-Humean argument for the subjectivity of values there is no reason to assume that even a classification with an evaluative aspect need not cut nature at its joints. The cost of this, however, is to accept the world contains more real features than those described by basic science. The nature of nature is more complex than that underpinned by reductionist or scientistic metaphysics. Reductionist naturalism should be replaced by relaxed naturalism.

In addition to the broadside of anti-psychiatric criticism, there are further reasons to question the validity of psychiatric classification. One source is internal criticism based on favouring a different kind of classification. One based on ideal types, on symptoms rather than syndromes or continuously varying quantities. Another is the complication raised by adding idiographic, by contrast with criterial or more generally nomothetic, factors.

To assess these I looked to resources drawn from the philosophy of science where debate about realism more generally has been more common. Two tests for realism within science are inference to the best explanation and inference to the cause. Either of these could apply to psychiatric taxonomy, but at the same time, arguments from Arthur Fine suggest that neither of these can provide an extra-theoretic perspective. For anyone sceptical of the underlying truth of scientific theories (or the reality of the underlying entities), neither test should be convincing because they are both question begging. This suggests that there is no theory-neutral test for the validity of psychiatric classification, no theory neutral way to prefer either zones of rarity or aetiological theory as the better measure of whether classification cuts nature at its joints.

Finally, I considered the question of the validity of narrative elements of so-called comprehensive diagnosis. The very idea of an individualistic element pulls against the paradigmatic validity of the Periodic Table that is based on general, criterial and nomothetic understanding. The strength of the Periodic Table lies in its ability to prescind from surface complexity to chart shared underlying structure. Individualistic understanding in comprehensive diagnosis, by contrast, stresses precisely the 'surface complexity': the individual features that constitute a subject's life. It is thus not surprising that it fails to meet the kind of tests that have been suggested by debate in the philosophy of science, but bearing in mind that the very vocabulary that is used to make sense of fellow humans and to chart the meaning and significance in individual lives is itself subject to overall critical scrutiny, there is a different kind of test for such understanding. This depends on making critical rational judgements of the plausibility not only of individual accounts, but also the very concepts used to frame them. This, however, is just an aspect of reason's longstanding obligation for self-critical scrutiny.

## Chapter 6

# The relation of evidence-based medicine and tacit knowledge in clinical judgement

## Plan of the chapter

1. **The presence of evidence-based medicine in psychiatry**

2. **Hume's challenge to induction**

3. **Responses to Hume**

   Hume's own response

   Mill's methods

   The consequences of Hume's problem and Mill's methods for RCTs and EBM

4. **The role of individual judgement in induction**

   A Wittgensteinian response to Hume's challenge to induction

5. **Conclusions**

This chapter examines the nature of evidence-based medicine as applied to psychiatry. At heart, evidence-based medicine (EBM) aims to codify how to base psychiatric diagnosis, and especially treatment and management, on evidence. EBM thus concerns how best to learn from collective experience. It makes substantial claims about which forms of evidence are more reliable, better guides to the truth of clinical judgement. How can those prescriptions be justified? Are they based on *a priori* reasoning or are they, themselves, evidence based? A clearer understanding of this question can be drawn from philosophical analysis of how experience can in general justify predictions about the future.

This chapter thus examines the Scottish philosopher David Hume's challenge to induction and contrasts his general sceptical conclusions with John Stuart Mill's concrete articulation of several methods of 'eliminative induction'. Hume's argument, whilst deceptively simple, suggests a fundamental difficulty in providing a rule-based justification for supporting general claims by empirical evidence.

The second section sets out Hume's own response to his own sceptical challenge and contrasts it with John Stuart Mill's methods of eliminative induction. Mill's methods appear to offer *a priori* support for the method of clinical trials. On careful inspection, however, they cannot be put into practice. Approximations of the methods can be applied, but only once judgements have already been made about plausible causal factors.

The fourth section re-examines, for a third and final time, Wittgenstein's analysis of rule following and argues that, properly understood, it helps undermine Hume's sceptical argument. Induction and deduction are of a piece in that both depend on individual and ultimately uncodifiable judgements.

Taken together these will help shed light on the assumptions that govern EBM. One important further conclusion will be that, underlying whatever explicit practical guidelines that can be offered, there is an ineliminable role for practical know-how or tacit knowledge.

## 1. **The presence of evidence-based medicine in psychiatry**

One of the biggest influences on contemporary medical practice in recent years, on both general medicine and on psychiatry, has been the rise of evidence-based medicine. As well as playing an increasingly explicit role in medical education and training, other signs of its influence include: the launch of the journals, such as *Evidence-Based Medicine,* published by the BMJ Publishing Group. In the UK, clinical guidelines are provided by the National Institute of Clinical Excellence, and the National Institute of Mental Health in England (NIMHE) is charged with 'supporting change in mental health and mental health services' again through practice guidelines. In the US, a similar organisation, National Institute of Mental Health (NIMH), has the aim of reducing mental illness based on research from both basic science and clinical studies. There has also been an increasing use of meta-reviews of evidence published by the international organisation the Cochrane Collaboration.

The influence of EBM has also been felt within psychiatry. There is, for example, a specific journal-*Evidence-Based Mental Health.* In 1997, John Geddes and Paul Harrison, two Oxford University psychiatrists, wrote an overview of the application of evidence-based medicine to psychiatry for the *British Journal of Psychiatry* called 'Closing the gap between research and practice'. In it, they give a very clear account of the motivation for adopting EBM.

The motivation runs as follows. There is, they argue, a 'knowledge gap' between the accurate information generally employed by clinicians and the decisions that they make partly on the basis of it. In other words, clinical decisions are underdetermined by the readily available (pre-EBM) evidence (the under determination of theory by data was discussed in Chapter 5). This is not to say that the decisions are therefore made arbitrarily. Instead, the gap is filled by other factors: 'the conceptual aetiological school to which we subscribe' and 'the combination of experience and habits which we accumulate' (Geddes and Harrison 1997: 220). However, these factors vary from clinician to clinician, which thus undermines the *inter-rater* reliability of diagnosis and treatment. Nor are they empirically tested guides. Hence, they reveal a need for better grounded evidence to guide diagnosis and treatment in the form of EBM.

What then is EBM? Geddes and Harrison say that it is the 'conscientious, explicit and judicious use of the current best evidence in making decisions about the care of individual patients' (Geddes and Harrison 1997: 220). The kind of evidence in question is that provided through clinical trials, but there are issues about how to assess or rank conflicting evidence. The paper asserts that randomised control trials (RCTs), or better still systematic reviews of RCTs, are the most reliable study design for the evaluation of treatments. However, because such trials are not always available, Geddes and Harrison, following widely accepted principles of EBM, suggest that there is a hierarchy of kinds of evidence that can also be pressed into service. It is as follows:

1 (a) Evidence from a meta-analysis of RCTs.

 (b) Evidence from at least one RCT.

2 (a) Evidence from at least one controlled study without randomization.

 (b) Evidence from at least one other quasi-experimental study.

3 Evidence from non-experimental descriptive studies, such as comparative studies, correlation studies and case-control studies.

4 Evidence from expert committee reports, or opinions and/or clinical experience of respected authorities.

This hierarchy has become well known as a cornerstone of EBM. It helps give substance to the very idea of EBM since, without some specific content to its prescriptions, the idea that medical treatment should be based on evidence of one sort or another is nothing new. The hierarchy suggests what is, in part at least, a rule-governed approach. All other things being equal,

'RCTs, or better still, systematic reviews of RCTs', are the most reliable study design for the evaluation of treatments. However, for many interventions, RCTs may not exist and the practitioner has to use evidence from the next level of the hierarchy. The practical importance of the hierarchy is that, when choosing between treatments, the clinician selects the intervention which is backed up by the best available evidence' (Geddes and Harrison 1997: 221).

The key feature of the hierarchy, and what makes EBM a radical idea, is that expert opinion and clinical judgement is placed at the bottom of the list and meta-analysis is placed at the top. (Of course, the hierarchy is taught to medical students with the full rhetorical force of teachers' expert opinion. But, properly understood, that opinion is like a ladder which the student 'must so to speak throw away …, after he has climbed up on it' (Wittgenstein 1929: 6.54).)

In fact, Geddes and Harrison stress that there are also non-algorithmic aspects of clinical judgement. After considering a hypothetical case they say 'The example makes it clear that interpretation of evidence and health care decisions are complex even when good quality evidence is available and EBM is adopted. Evidence is helpful but not sufficient for medical decision making: the key aspect of EBM is that it ensures the best use is made of *available* evidence' (Geddes and Harrison 1997: 222). However, like the discussion of the role of the Four Principles of medical ethics discussed in Chapter 2, whilst the best accounts of the use of the EBM hierarchy might stress a role for uncodified but skilled judgements alongside what is codified, these elements can be forgotten in practice.

I argued in Chapter 2 that, in the case of medical ethics, the stress on codified ethical judgement resulted from a mistaken assumption that ethical principles provided the only resource for *disciplining* ethical judgements (even though, according to the Four Principles approach, such judgement is *not* determined by principles alone). The reason in this case is that what makes EBM powerful seems to pull in the opposite direction from any use of skilled individual judgement. The status of scientific medicine seems to be underpinned by an objective and impersonal scientific method constituted in part by reliance on, and application of, evidence drawn from RCTs above all else.

There is a similar tension between explicit statements of the role of judgement and implicit emphasis on the importance of rule-governed procedures in another influential, general statement of the principles of EBM. In their book, *Evidence-Based Medicine: How to practice and teach EBM*, David Sackett, Sharon Straus, Scott Richardson, William Rosenberg, and Brian Haynes define it as follows: 'Evidence-based medicine is the integration of best research evidence with clinical expertise and patient values' (Sackett *et al.* 2000).

This is a surprising definition. Normally, the focus of EBM is on the first element of that tripartite division: best research evidence. Sackett *et al.* widen their definition to include two further aspects: expertise and values. They give a further brief preliminary sketch of each as follows:

> By *best research evidence* we mean clinically relevant research … New evidence from clinical research and treatments both invalidates previously accepted diagnostic tests and treatments and replaces them with new ones that are more powerful, more accurate, more efficacious and safer.
>
> By *clinical expertise* we mean the ability to use our clinical skills and past experience to rapidly identify each patient's unique health state and diagnosis, their individual risks and benefits of potential interventions, and their personal values and expectations
>
> By *patient values* we mean the unique preferences, concerns and expectations each patient brings to a clinical encounter and which must be integrated into clinical decisions if they are to serve the patient. (Sackett *et al.* 2000: 3)

Two preliminary points are worth making about this substantial overall definition. First, it looks to be a definition of what would normally be taken to be, not EBM as such but, something that should be based on it: best clinical practice, perhaps, or clinical judgement. The wider definition is perhaps best interpreted as a definition of medicine that is evidence based, as well as, for example, values based.

Secondly, although Sackett *et al.* stress the role of clinical expertise and patient values in the first pages of their book, the rest of the book concerns research evidence exclusively. So one reaction to Sackett's book and the tripartite distinction is to conclude that judgement plays a role only in the second and third element. In the rest of this chapter, I aim to show that that is a mistaken view.

At its most abstract, evidence-based medicine is a codification of how best to learn from experience. But how can its ranking of forms of evidence be, itself, justified? Because it concerns how past experience should guide future practice, it belongs in a tradition of methodological prescriptions from the philosophy of science, which can be seen as responses, spread over 300 years, to David Hume's challenge to justify induction. By reviewing briefly both Hume's challenge and his own solution, and John Stuart Mill's methods of eliminative induction a century later, the status of EBM and the role of judgement within it can be pin pointed.

## 2. **Hume's challenge to induction**

Hume's challenge to induction is contained in his *Enquiries Concerning Human Understanding and Concerning the Principles of Morals* Section iv (Hume (1748) 1975). He starts his argument with the bold claim that all the objects of human reason can be divided between relations of ideas and matters of fact. This distinction, generally known as 'Hume's Fork', sets up the contrast that will be important between the status of knowledge claims, which can be arrived at through deductive demonstration and those for which a merely inductive warrant can be provided.

It is worth noting, briefly, two features that characterise the distinction:

- Truths that comprise relations of ideas can be determined to hold purely through examination of the constituent ideas rather than looking outwards, as it were, at how things stand in the world. Thus, they do not depend on, or presuppose, any existence claims. Thus, the claim that the square of the hypotenuse of a triangle is equal to the sum of the squares of the other two sides is a truth that is independent of whether there are any right-angled triangles in the universe.

- The negation of truths that comprise relations of ideas produces claims that could not have been true and cannot be 'distinctly conceived by the mind'. By contrast, the negation of matters of fact could have been true and thus can be so conceived. This amounts to saying that relations of ideas express necessary, rather than just contingent truths.

A distinction of this sort has been influential throughout empiricist philosophy. Consider the following three binary distinctions between kinds of truth:

- epistemological: *a priori* versus *a posteriori*;
- metaphysical: necessary versus contingent;
- semantic: analytic versus synthetic.

These are three distinct ways to classify truths—such as true statements or true beliefs—according to whether, respectively:

- they can be known independently of experience (*a priori*);
- they must be true (this is sometimes put by saying they are truths that hold in all, rather than merely some, 'possible worlds') (neessary);
- their truth is merely a matter of their meaning rather than a combination of meaning and worldly fact (analytic).

One appealing assumption has been that these different ways of sorting truths all sort truths into the same sets. Thus, all truths that can be known *a priori* (that is, without experience) are necessarily true and their truth is fixed by the concepts used to frame them (they are analytically true, true in virtue of their meaning). Equally, all truths that require experience to be known and are, thus, *a posteriori*, are also contingent and synthetic (their truth requires both a contribution from their meaning and from the world).

There are also *prima facie* plausible arguments for the alignment of these distinctions. For example, if a truth can be known *a priori* then one does not need to know which 'possible world' one inhabits in order to know its truth.

That is, one does not need to know which of all the possible ways things might have been is actually the case. Experience, however, teaches us which of the many possible worlds we actually live in. Thus, if a truth can be known without knowing which possible world one inhabits then this must be because it holds in all possible worlds and is thus a necessary truth. Furthermore, it seems plausible that it must be analytic for the following reason. If its truth does not depend on a contribution from the way a specific possible world is it seems plausible that it does not depend on any worldly contribution at all. If so, its truth must be fixed by its meaning alone.

Despite these arguments, the neat alignment of truths has also come under attack. Immanuel Kant (1724–1804) argued that there were synthetic truths that could be known *a priori* including mathematics (Kant 1929: 52–54). His main argument for this was that no examination of the concepts expressed by the words 'seven', 'five' and 'plus' could yield the concept expressed by 'twelve'. That took a further leap of understanding. Thus, mathematics had to be synthetic, rather than analytic. More recently, the logician Saul Kripke argued that some *a posteriori* truths are, nevertheless, necessary (such as the discovery that water is $H_2O$), whilst the American philosopher W.V.O. Quine (1908–2000) attacked the assumption that the distinctions are actually well founded and clear cut (Quine 1961; Kripke 1980).

What matters here, however, is that drawing the distinction between relations of ideas and matters of fact allows Hume to focus the issue of the foundations of matters of fact. (If the distinctions do not align or are not even firm, this will not solve the general problem Hume raises for justifying empirical knowledge. It merely changes the form it takes because there ceases to be a clear contrast between fallible *a posteriori* reasoning and the supposedly certain *a priori* and deductive reasoning.)

Having drawn the distinction, Hume then focuses his attention on the status of knowledge of matters of fact. In fact, the focus is narrower still: on knowledge of what lies 'beyond the present testimony of our senses, or the record of our memory' (Hume (1748) 1975: 26). Thus, he does not here investigate the status of direct observational knowledge of particular matters of fact—knowledge made available by opening one's eyes to the world (such as in a physical examination)—or even memory of such particular facts.

On the one hand, this sets up an implicit contrast between observation and induction. The latter appears less reliable than the former. Indeed, induction in general can never have a stronger justification than observation in general because inductive inferences take observations as their premises. But on further reflection, observation reports are typically laden with theory. They can, in individual cases, thus be overturned on the basis of enough inductive counter-evidence. (The other implicit contrast is between induction and deduction. This latter contrast will play an important role towards the end of the chapter.)

Hume suggests that inductive reasoning is founded on the relation of cause and effect. It is this relation that underpins reasoning beyond our direct observations and binds unobserved facts to observed facts. 'Were there nothing to bind them together, the inference would be entirely precarious' (Hume (1748) 1975: 27). However, Hume goes on to question what grounds our knowledge of cause–effect relations. He argues that this cannot be a piece of *a priori* reasoning and is instead based on our experience. He argues both that cause–effect relations concern separate events and, thus, no amount of inspection of the cause–event can yield knowledge of what effect it will lead to, and also that the negation of cause–effect relations does not produce any logical contradiction or a state of affairs that cannot be distinctly conceived. Having cleared the ground in this way, Hume goes on to discuss how experience, rather than *a priori* demonstration, can ground our knowledge of cause–effect relations.

Section IV, part II of the *Enquiries* contains the sceptical discussion of induction. Hume begins by asking, on the assumption (for which he has just argued) that the foundation of our knowledge of matters of fact (aside from the case of direct perception) is knowledge of cause–effect relations, what underpins our knowledge of that relation? His answer is experience. This seems like a good answer and in everyday contexts would mark the end point of inquiry, but Hume, like a good philosopher, then asks a further question: 'what is the foundation of all conclusions from experience?' (Hume (1748) 1975: 32). He suggests that he will argue that our knowledge of matters of fact is not founded on *reasoning* from past experience.

Hume takes as an example the connection between the sensible or observational properties of bread and its 'secret power' to provide nourishment. Experience can play a direct role in establishing that there has been such a connection in particular cases in the past, but how can experience underpin the extension of a more general connection 'to future times, and to other objects'?

> These two propositions are far from being the same, I have found that such an object has always been attended with such an effect, and I foresee, that other objects, which are, in appearance similar, will be attended with similar effects. I shall allow, if you please, that the one proposition may justly be inferred from the other: I know, in fact, that it always is inferred. But if you insist that the inference is made by a chain of reasoning, I desire you to produce that reasoning. (Hume (1748) 1975: 34)

Hume goes on to argue that inductive inferences cannot be demonstrative because their negations make good sense. Bread might not nourish in the future even though it has in the past. The course of nature could (logically possibly) change. Thus, there seems no prospect of a deductive defence of induction because it would be too strong, but on the other hand, inductive defences of induction also appear hopeless because circular. Hume suggests that empirical reasoning:

> proceed(s) upon the supposition that the future will be conformable to the past. To endeavour, therefore, the proof of this last supposition by probable arguments, or arguments regarding existence (i.e. inductive arguments about matters of fact), must be evidently going in a circle, and taking that for granted, which is the very point in question. (Hume (1748) 1975: 35–6)

So stepping back from the details of Hume's argument we can set out the problem as follows. Suppose that the premise is that all bread previously tested has been nourishing and the conclusion is that all future bread will be nourishing. Hume's challenge is to explain what form of inference justifies the conclusion. The natural suggestion is that experience grounds the *rule* of inference, as well as the *premiss* (in this case that all bread previously tested has been nourishing). It does this because of the more general piece of direct experiential knowledge that correlations between (in this case what Hume calls) 'sensible qualities' and 'secret powers' have held over time. This general experiential finding is then used to ground the inference from past to future in the specific bread case, but as Hume points out, using experience to ground the rule itself presupposes that very rule as an inference. Why should the fact that such correlations have held in the past support the claim that they will hold in the future unless an inductive inference is justified here as well?

Hume says:

> When a man says, I have found, in all past instances, such sensible qualities conjoined with such secret powers: And when he says, Similar sensible qualities will always be conjoined with similar secret powers, he is not guilty of a tautology, nor are these propositions in any respect the same. You say that the one proposition is an inference from the other. But you must confess that the inference is not intuitive; neither is it demonstrative: Of what nature is it then? To say it is experimental, is begging the question. For all inferences from experience suppose, as their foundation, that the future will resemble the past ... It is impossible, therefore, that any arguments from experience can prove this resemblance of the past to the future; since all these arguments are founded on the supposition of that resemblance. (Hume (1748) 1975: 36–7)

This passage suggests the following alternatives. For experience to yield a principle which will underpin reasoning from observed to unobserved cases we need an argument of the following sort:

- *Premiss 1*: Correlations have held in the past (observed cases).
- *Conclusion*: Correlations will hold in the future (unobserved cases).

Now by itself this argument is not demonstrative or deductive: it is not a valid argument. If experience of the stability of past correlations is to justify the claim that they will continue to be stable, it does this in virtue of an *inductive* inference, but that was the very rule that this argument was supposed to justify, rather than presuppose.

On the other hand, Hume suggests that such arguments presuppose that the future will resemble the past. Now putting aside the details of how it resembles it, if this were true, inductive arguments would be successful, in the sense of leading to the truth, but how is this fact supposed to help justify those arguments? The obvious answer is that if this is introduced as a second premiss, the argument becomes a valid demonstrative argument:

- ◆ *Premiss 1*: Correlations have held in the past (observed cases).
- ◆ *Premiss 2*: The future resembles the past (unobserved cases resemble observed cases).
- ◆ *Conclusion*: Correlations will hold in the future (unobserved cases).

However, if it is to underwrite a true conclusion, this valid argument requires the truth of the second premiss that is, as Hume points out, not a necessary truth or a truth that can be arrived at demonstratively. It might have been false. If that is true then it seems to be based on empirical findings, but if so, it would require a further inductive argument to justify it. So in either case there appears to be no non-circular argument for inductive reasoning from past experience to future cases.

Hume's argument suggests the following worry. If we make a knowledge claim about unobserved events on the basis of observed events we open ourselves up to the challenge of providing grounds. Now there are first and second moves available to us. We can justify our claim about the *unobserved* by citing our experience of the *observed*. Hume can then challenge us to say how exactly that experience of what has been *observed* has a bearing on what has so far *not been observed*. We can then say (as our second justificatory move) that we have more general experience (that is, we have *observed* the following) that *observed* matters have always (in the past) been a good guide to initially *unobserved* but subsequently observed matters.

Prior to reading Hume, this looks to discharge the burden of providing grounds for our original claim, but he suggests that this second justificatory claim only works if we can take it for granted that past experience is a good guide to future experience or that what is observed is a good guide to what is unobserved, and that is just what he is challenging us to justify. At this point we have apparently no further arguments to make and the chain of justifications comes unstitched backwards from here. If we cannot justify induction in general, we cannot justify it in the particular case at hand. Thus, we cannot say what the relevance of our past experience is to our claim about the unobserved and, thus, we cannot justify that supposed knowledge claim. Therefore, we must admit that we do not know it, despite our pre-philosophical inclinations.

Now this may seem to be a merely philosophical problem, but one of the emphases of the rise of EBM in psychiatry is to make assessment of evidence both as explicit and sophisticated as possible. Thus, it would be, at the very least, an embarrassment to that project if there were no answer to what seems to be a straightforward argument about the role of inductive evidence as a whole.

## 3. Responses to Hume

Reading Hume's sceptical attack on induction can, like any piece of philosoph-ical scepticism, lead to a kind of disorientation. On the one hand, the argu-ment appears to be persuasive. The premises seem to be true and the argument valid, but on the other, the conclusion appears to be intolerable. Forming judgements about the future on the basis of past experience appears to be at the heart of rational activity, not least scientific medicine. Therefore, how can it not be justifiable?

### Hume's own response

Hume himself suggests two related kinds of response to his own challenge. One response is to emphasise a custom-based or anthropological perspective. As a matter of fact, Hume stresses, we both do and practically must form just the sort of inferences he has criticised:

> Custom is that principle, by which this correspondence has been effected; so neces-sary to the subsistence of our species, and the regulation of our conduct, in every circumstance and occurrence of human life. Had not the presence of an object, instantly excited the idea of those objects, commonly conjoined with it, all our knowl-edge must have been limited to the narrow sphere of our memory and senses; and we should never have been able to adjust means to ends, or employ our natural powers, either to the producing of good, or avoiding of evil. (Hume (1748) 1975: 55)

This response is not very satisfactory by itself, however. After all, Hume's sceptical attack is against the idea that the custom or practice of forming induction judgements is *justified*. Emphasising its centrality to human prac-tices does not address that point and show how the practice is justified, as well as being central. The threat is, precisely, that a centrally important practice might be unjustified. That is why the scepticism is so disorientating.

Hume's second response is to suggest that the argument he has given serves as a kind of *reductio ad absurdum*, not for forming empirical beliefs through induction, but of the kind of deductive argument used against it. Both views are expressed in this passage:

> [T]his operation of the mind, by which we infer like effects from like causes, and vice versa, is so essential to the subsistence of all human creatures, it is not probable, that it could be trusted to the fallacious deductions of our reason, which is slow in its operations; appears not, in any degree, during the first years of infancy; and at best is, in every age and period of human life, extremely liable to error and mistake. (Hume (1748) 1975: 55)

Thus, Hume suggests that, given the centrality of inductive inference, the sceptical argument framed as a piece of deductive reasoning counts against deduction rather than induction. Although that might not seem a very promising idea, by examining Wittgenstein's analysis of rule following towards the end of this chapter, I will aim to show that it does help to defuse Humean scepticism.

Recent responses to Hume within broadly Anglo-American philosophy can be divided into two distinct kinds. They either attempt to defuse Hume's argument and thus show that induction can, in fact, be justified (this is the approach taken within the branch of philosophy called 'epistemology'). They attempt to sidestep the problem by outlining methods for theory choice in science that do not presuppose an answer to Hume's scepticism (this approach is more common within 'philosophy of science'). There is also a hint of each of these responses in Hume's dual approach outlined above.

One modern element of an *epistemological* attempt to defuse Humean inductive scepticism is to deny the assumption that a justification for knowledge has itself to be known. As long as the justification is *true*, that is enough for ground level knowledge. With this in place, whilst there may be a kind of scepticism about whether the justifications for ground level knowledge claims are true, mere ignorance of this question is not enough to undermine the ground level knowledge. (For further discussion of this see Fulford *et al.* 2006: 433–62.)

An influential starting point for the second approach in the philosophy of science is Sir Karl Popper's Falsificationism (Popper 1959). Popper argues that science does not need to establish the truth of theories on the basis of evidence. Rather, it aims to use evidence to refute or falsify theories and thus to reject them as false. Although Falsificationism is a popular account of science among scientists, in its pure form it cannot underpin EBM as conventionally understood because it does not allow any positive inductive support for theories or, in this case, treatment choices. Unfalsified theories retain the status merely of guesses for strict Falsificationism. Nevertheless, it will be useful to highlight the role of skilled judgement in EBM by looking at one of the philosophical precursors of Falsificationism: Mill's methods of eliminative induction. Afterwards, I will return to consider the role that tacit knowledge might have in a broadly Humean account of EBM by looking, once more in this book, to Wittgenstein's analysis of rule following.

## Mill's methods

Whilst Hume's general argument raises doubts about the rationality of inductive inferences, Mill's methods of eliminative induction appear to provide a model of a clear cut and justified approach. What is more, one of them seems to lie at the heart of EBM because it lies at the heart of clinical trials. Nevertheless, closer attention to them suggests a gulf between principle and practice which can only be filled by something akin to a solution to, or at least accommodation with, Hume's problem of induction.

In his *System of Logic*, John Stuart Mill (1806–73) outlines five experimental methods that he suggests can underpin experimental inquiry. These are:

- the method of agreement;
- the method of difference;
- the joint method of agreement and difference;
- the method of residues;
- the method of concomitant variations.

In fact, because the last three are based on the first two, I will discuss only the methods of agreement and difference.

The method of agreement is as follows:

> If two or more instances of the phenomenon under investigation have only one circumstance in common, the circumstance in which alone all the instances agree, is the cause (or effect) of the given phenomenon ...
>
> If our object be to discover the effects of an agent A, we must procure A in some set of ascertained circumstances, as A B C, and having noted the effects produced, compare them with the effect of the remaining circumstances B C, when A is absent. If the effect of A B C is a b c, and the effect of B C, b c, it is evident that the effect of A is a. (Mill 1970: 255)

As a model of clinical research, the method of agreement is of limited use. One example that approximates to it is the work done by John Snow (1813–1858), a member of the Royal College of Surgeons of England. After an outbreak of cholera in 1854, Snow investigated the spread of the disease by mapping its victims in London. He discovered that the key common element in each case was that the victims had drunk water from a particular well. After officials followed Snow's advice to remove the handle of the Broad Street pump, the epidemic was contained.

This is, however, only an approximate application of the method of agreement. The method proper requires that the only condition which a variety of experimental cases have in common turns out to be the cause of the (controlled for) effect in question or, vice versa, is the effect of the cause in question. Clearly, the practical difficulties of picking a trial sample of items which were alike in only one respect would be enormous, but on further reflection this is really a principled problem because there is no limit to the number of (e.g. relational) properties that an individual (a human being or simply a thing) has. All human subjects, for example, share the property of being in the earth's gravitational field, of being in this part of the galaxy, of being bigger than a pea and so on.

The method of difference is a better model for clinical research. It is defined thus:

> If an instance in which the phenomenon under investigation occurs, and an instance in which it does not occur, have every circumstance in common save one, that one occurring only in the former; the circumstances in which alone the two instances differ, is the effect, or the cause, or an indispensable part of the cause, of the phenomenon. It is inherent in the peculiar character of the Method of Difference that the nature of the combinations which it requires is much more strictly defined than in the Method of Agreement. The two instances which are to be compared with one another must be exactly similar in all circumstances except the one which we are attempting to investigate: they must be in the relation of A B C and B C, or of a b c and b c. (Mill 1970: 256)

Mill suggests that the conditions for this method are rarely spontaneously met in nature since they require that two circumstances are exactly alike except for one feature, but they can be met experimentally. Mill suggests introducing a new phenomenon to a situation—perhaps by physically moving a substance or adding a chemical to another chemical—yields just this sort of pair of circumstances. He warns, however, that the method of bringing about a change might itself constitute an important difference from the initial circumstance:

> There is one doubt, indeed, which may remain in some cases of this description; the effect may have been produced not by the change, but by the means employed to produce the change. The possibility, however, of this last supposition generally admits of being conclusively tested by other experiments. (Mill 1970: 257)

He gives a concrete example:

> If a bird is taken from a cage, and instantly plunged into carbonic gas, the experimentalist may be fully assured (at all events after one or two repetitions) that no circumstance capable of causing suffocation had supervened in the interim, except the change from immersion in the atmosphere to immersion in carbonic gas. (Mill 1970: 257)

The method of difference also forms a plausible model of much clinical research. Clinical trials are generally contrastive. The effects of a drug on one trial group, for example, are compared with the effects of no such treatment (in fact, generally a placebo) on another 'control' group. If the one group is treated in the same way as the other in all respects other than the administration of the drug, then the subsequent differences are the causal result of the drug treatment. (I will return to the differences between such trials and the method of difference shortly.)

So, what exactly do these methods achieve? Mill describes them as methods of *eliminative* induction, which contrasts with the Humean idea of enumerative induction—building up generalisations from particular (past) cases. Mill's methods are negative: they aim at eliminating conditions as irrelevant to cause–effect relations. Therefore, they resemble Popper's Falsificationism (described above).

The method of agreement is a method of eliminating conditions from a list of conditions that are necessary for another condition—an effect, for example. (Any conditions that are *not* present when the effect in question occurs cannot be *necessary* conditions of that effect.) The method can also be used to determine sufficient conditions. In this case, one looks for those conditions that are *never* present when an effect is absent. (If a condition is present when an effect is absent, then it cannot be sufficient for that effect.) Thus, one slowly eliminates conditions from a list of potential sufficient conditions.

This much is a matter of definition of what 'necessary' and 'sufficient' mean. The method is thus, in one sense, trivial. It is the unpacking of the consequence of the definition of those terms. This, however, underpins its validity. (Whilst I will not discuss it here, there is also at least a connection between the concepts of necessity and sufficiency, and that of cause, albeit not an unproblematic one. One account suggests that a cause is an insufficient, but necessary element of an unnecessary, but sufficient condition (Mackie 1993).)

The method of difference provides a way of eliminating conditions that are not sufficient for an effect from some overall circumstance which is sufficient; that is, when the effect is present. (Any factors that are present when an effect in question is not present cannot themselves be sufficient for that effect.) Now there may be many different sufficient conditions, but the method of difference is a way of paring down some complex combination that is itself sufficient to find out which parts of it are not sufficient. Again, this follows from the definition of the terms involved.

Mill's methods provide models for determining causal connections, models that can be arrived at *a priori*. (Strictly, Mill's methods concern logical relations of necessity and sufficiency. The connection between these notions and causality is a matter of debate, but nearly everyone agrees that causality is related to necessity and sufficiency.) They are, however, overly simplified models of empirical research. They cannot provide an *a priori* argument for the EBM evidence hierarchy.

Recall the criticism of the method of agreement above. It is impossible to ensure that different complex circumstances have nothing (except a condition under scrutiny) in common. Likewise in the case of the method of difference, it is impossible to ensure that two different circumstances are identical in all but one respect. (If they are distinct, are they in different places, for example?) But it is practically possible to ensure that nothing *causally relevant* is the same in the former case or different in the latter case. This suggests that Mill's methods cannot play a foundational role, a role that presupposes no other causal knowledge. Rather, the role of Mill's methods lies within a background of other fallible prior scientific beliefs about what causes what. They are a further constraint on our causal knowledge.

A further way of bringing this out is to consider Mill's use of letters to label different conditions (antecedent conditions A, B, C and succeeding conditions a, b, c). Mill begins his discussion of the methods in the following way:

> We shall denote antecedents by the large letters of the alphabet, and the consequents corresponding to them by the small. Let A, then, be an agent or cause, and let the object of our inquiry be to ascertain what are the effects of this cause. (Mill 1970: 253–4)

One of his critics, the philosopher of science William Whewell, objected to just this way of setting up the problem:

> Upon these methods, the obvious thing to remark is, that they take for granted the very thing which is most difficult to discover, the reduction of the phenomena to formulae such as are here presented to us. (Whewell 1849: 44)

Mill simply assumes that we already possess, when searching for causal factors, a complete description which captures all the causally relevant factors (causes A, B and C, and effects a, b and c). Given this, then elimination of irrelevant factors is comparatively easy, but from where did this vocabulary arise?

As recent work on the problem of induction has emphasised, one cannot simply read off correct inductive generalisations form the world. One argument for this is Nelson Goodman's New Riddle of Induction (Goodman 1983). Goodman invents two new predicates (or adjectives): 'grue' and 'bleen', where 'grue' means green until some time in the future, say the year 2020 and blue afterwards, and 'bleen' means blue until then and green afterwards. Now the predicate 'grue' could be applied to all the healthy grass so far observed as far as past evidence is concerned, as could 'green', but the grass is either grue or green, not both. (It either will or will not turn blue in 2020.) So what is it that supports our projecting its greenness into the future not its grueness? What is it that makes a predicate projectable? (Note that the quick response that grue and bleen are time-dependent, whilst green and blue are not is not decisive. A supporter of grue and bleen will point out that 'green' means grue before 2020 and bleen afterwards, and thus is time dependent itself.)

Both of these points can be translated into the context of mental health to raise yet further practical difficulties. Establishing conditions as the same in all but one respect (in the method of agreement) or different in all but one (method of difference) is difficult enough in the case of physical medicine, but establishing these cases for psychiatric conditions is even more difficult. To mention just one reason: psychiatric symptoms are rarely present in isolation, but are combined in ways that are not exactly repeated between different patients. Weakening the requirement to take account of only causally relevant features (as mentioned above) will not help in this case because the prior judgement of just what is and is not causally relevant in psychiatry is far from settled.

Likewise, the prospect of reducing a description of the state of individuals' mental lives to the letters illustratively used by Mill seems particularly artificial and unlikely in the case of mental health. This is not to say that there is no chance of a valid description of psychiatric symptoms. That remains a major aim both of psychiatric theorising and of revisions to psychiatric taxonomy (see Chapter 5). However, Mill's use of letters is supposed to be an unproblematic basis for a foundational method of inductive reasoning not part of a fallible and holistic approach to scientific psychiatry.

## The consequences of Hume's problem and Mill's methods for RCTs and EBM

The purpose of going back to Hume's original challenge to induction and Mill's methods of eliminative induction is to shed light on the methods that underpin evidence-based medicine. Insofar as EBM is based on contrastive clinical trials, then it inherits the dilemma that faces Mill's method of difference. If the method could be precisely applied, then it would possess an *a priori* validity, but given that it cannot be, then its application depends on a prior judgement of the causally relevant factors. This is, of course, addressed in part by randomization, but even that presupposes a prior judgement as to what factors are relevant for randomization: typically age (within limits), gender, socio-economic background and so on. (It is not the case that *every* factor is randomized.)

Secondly, although I have followed Mill in describing the methods as methods of logic and interpreted this as an *a priori* and analytic matter, Mill himself slips into an enumerative style of induction in one of the quotes above. He says: 'If a bird is taken from a cage, and instantly plunged into carbonic gas, the experimentalist may be fully assured (*at all events after one or two repetitions*) that no circumstance capable of causing suffocation had supervened in the interim' (Mill 1970: 257, italics added). However, repetition has no place in the methods proper. Once Mill admits that actually testing for intervening factors is a matter of repeating the experiment, he both moves closer to the methods of actual clinical trials, but away from an algorithmic and logical model. Such repetitions have argumentative force only in the context of Humean custom or, as I will stress, practised judgement.

Finally, in accord with Whewell's criticism of Mill, the experimental set up of a clinical trial is based on a particular description of putative causal factors and putative effects. Thus, the test in any application of the method of difference, or any RCT based on this method, presupposes the validity of the vocabulary used in the descriptions of the set up. This point is made in a recent paper by the Zurich-based psychiatrist, Thomas Maier:

> The evidence-based approach to individual cases is critically dependent on the validity of diagnoses. This is an axiomatic assumption of EBM, which is rarely analysed or scrutinised in detail. If in a concrete case, no diagnosis could be attributed, the case would not be amenable to EBM, and no evidence could support decisions in such cases. If the diagnosis is wrong, or—even more intricate—if cases labelled with a defined diagnosis are still not homogenous enough to be comparable in relevant aspects, EBM will provide useless results. (Maier 2006: 327)

Thus, there is a direct connection between the debate discussed in Chapter 5 and this one. If the validity of psychiatric classification is called into question, this calls into question the ability of clinicians to bring to bear the right evidence. At the same time, classifications are based on evidence:

> Kendell & Jablensky (2003) have also addressed the issue of diagnostic entities in a recent paper, and concluded that the validity of psychiatric diagnoses is limited. They analysed whether diagnostic entities are sufficiently separable from each other and from normality by *zones of rarity*. This is not the case, however; mental diagnoses are often overlapping (Welsby 1999; Cooper 2004); they shift over time in the same patient, and several similar diagnoses can be present in the same patient (co-morbidity). Not surprisingly, diagnosis alone is a poor predictor of outcome (Williams and Garner 2002). Acknowledging this haziness of diagnoses, one realizes the problems arising, when trying to match individual cases to empirical evidence. When even the presence of a (correctly assessed) diagnosis does not assure comparability to other cases with the same diagnosis, empirical evidence is highly questionable (Harari 2001). (Maier 2006: 327–8)

Thus, addressing the validity of diagnosis and addressing the nature of best inductive and evidential practice are two aspects of a single broader project concerned with the status of psychiatric judgement. In both, there is a key role for judgement about how the evidence is best interpreted. A further clue to the nature of this judgement will be explored in the next section on the role of tacit and individual judgement in psychiatry. This will also help provide a response to Hume's challenge to induction.

## 4. The role of individual judgement in induction

On the face of it, the rise of evidence-based medicine suggests the increasing role of codified expertise within medical practice. As described above, at the heart of EBM is a hierarchy of forms of evidence with meta-analysis of randomized control trials at the top. The suggestion is that clinicians should follow this hierarchy in assessing the evidence base for proposed treatments. Both the very existence of a written hierarchy and the fact it places expert clinical judgement at the bottom, suggests that scientific judgement about evidence can be codified. Despite that appearance, EBM merely disguises the role of uncodified clinical skill. I will summarise two further reasons for this before reiterating how an argument derived from Wittgenstein and already deployed in earlier chapters places uncodified skilled judgement at the heart of concept application, and thus psychiatric diagnosis and treatment. This same argument will also help provide a response to Hume's sceptical challenge to any form of inductive reasoning, but to begin I will outline the role of tacit knowledge in EBM.

First, there is a gap between published research and a specific case presented clinically. Whilst the EBM hierarchy suggests that judgements about the respective merits of published trials (or, preferably, the meta-analysis of trials) can, *prima facie*, be codified, the *relevance* of such trials to specific cases is not itself encoded in the trials themselves. This claim can be defended using an argument based on the possibility of a regress. Suppose that the relevance of a particular trial to a particular kind of client group were included in an introduction to it, or in a further guide to published trials, it would still be necessary to make a judgement about whether any particular subject belonged to that client group. Is that group and data about it relevant in this case? Whatever general claims are codified about a client group, the specific question of whether they apply to a particular subject will always arise on pain of infinite regress of further codifications. Assessing whether a published study applies to the case at hand is a further judgement of the relative similarities, since every subject is like every other in some respects and unlike them in others.

Secondly, as I have described elsewhere, meta-analyses of clinical trials may disguise but still presuppose the prior exercise of tacit skill in judgement

(Thornton 2006). Trials are experiments and, as such, depend on the skills on which such experiments depend. To take just one aspect, as the sociologist of knowledge Harry Collins argues, scientific replication turns on balancing two opposing factors (Collins 1985). To add epistemic weight, a new trial must be sufficiently unlike, but not too unlike, a previous result. A second EEG reading on the same experimental apparatus moments after the first reading is made adds little extra evidential force. A 'reading' based instead on the arrangement of tea leaves in a cup is too unlike the first to count as successful replication. A useful replication must compromise between these two extremes of similarity and dissimilarity. The judgement of what counts as sufficiently similar but different to be a replication cannot be specified in general context-free terms. It is, instead, a matter of skilled judgement in context. Like the other skills involved in teasing results out of real empirical settings, however, it becomes disguised once data is summarised in final meta-analytic terms.

There is also a deeper non-empirical reason for insisting that even factual judgements rest on an uncodified element. Even when a form of judgement can be codified as the application of a principle or rule, the application of the rule still depends on an element of uncodified skill. The argument for this claim derives from the later Wittgenstein and has been introduced in Chapter 2 (in partial support for the claim that value judgements need not be codified to be objective) and Chapter 4 (to show that meanings cannot be reduced either to internal mental representations or to ongoing production in conversation). Here, I will re-present the argument at length to show its role in placing good judgement at the heart of psychiatric practice. It will also underpin a final response to Hume's scepticism about induction.

The Wittgensteinian argument is drawn from his discussion of rule following in central sections of his *Philosophical Investigations*. A key example, described in Chapter 2, is continuing a mathematical series (such as 'add 2'), which looks at first to be completely specified (there seems to be no room for judgement). To tease out the gap between the codification and actual practice, however, Wittgenstein considers how one can ascribe understanding of the series to another person, or, relatedly, how one can successfully teach it to them, but the moral applies also to the first person case.

One problem is that, however many numbers a student may have successfully 'processed' (they have moved from 72 to 74 to 76, and so on), there is an open-ended continuation yet to be negotiated. Given the infinite number of variations in principle available at some higher number (for example, responding to the instruction 'add 2' by continuing 996, 998, 1000, but then 1004, 1008, and so forth), it may seem epistemically risky to ascribe shared understanding of the correct continuation on the basis of any amount of finite past practice as it will still comprise a vanishingly small proportion of the total. Indeed, as a mere induction, it would be risky:

> Let us return to our example (§143). Now—judged by the usual criteria—the pupil has mastered the series of natural numbers. Next we teach him to write down other series of cardinal numbers and get him to the point of writing down series of the form
>
> 0, n, 2n, 3n, etc.
>
> at an order of the form '+ n'; so at the order '+ 1' he writes down the series of natural numbers—Let us suppose we have done exercises and given him tests up to 1000. Now we get the pupil to continue a series (say + 2) beyond 1000–and he writes 1000, 1004, 1008, 1012. We say to him: 'Look what you've done!'—He doesn't understand. We say: 'You were meant to add *two*: look how you began the series!'—He answers: 'Yes, isn't it right? I thought that was how I was *meant* to do it.'—Or suppose he pointed to the series and said: 'But I went on in the same way.'—It would now be no use to say: 'But can't you see …?'—and repeat the old examples and explanations.— In such a case we might say, perhaps: It comes natural to this person to understand our order with our explanations as we should understand the order: 'Add 2 up to 1000, 4 up to 2000, 6 up to 3000 and so on.' (Wittgenstein 1953: §185)

By considering a student who mistakenly, but deliberately, follows a 'bent rule' that deviates from the correct continuation of '+ 2' at 1000, Wittgenstein raises the question of what keeps normal students on the right tracks. This example naturally prompts the thought that more was needed to rule out potential misunderstandings and that it would have been possible to exclude misunderstandings through more exact specification. In a passage which swaps from the third person case to the first person, Wittgenstein argues that that is not helpful:

> 'But this initial segment of a series obviously admitted of various interpretations (e.g. by means of algebraic expressions) and so you must first have chosen *one* such inter- pretation.'—Not at all. A doubt was possible in certain circumstances. But that is not to say that I did doubt, or even could doubt. (There is something to be said, which is connected with this, about the psychological 'atmosphere' of a process.) So it must have been intuition that removed this doubt?—If intuition is an inner voice—how do I know *how* I am to obey it? And how do I know that it doesn't mislead me? For if it can guide me right, it can   also guide me wrong. ((Intuition an unnecessary shuffle.)) If you have to have an intuition in order to develop the series 1 2 3 4 … you must also have one in order to develop the series 2 2 2 2 … (Wittgenstein 1953: §213–4)

The first comment here is a reminder that very often one has no doubt about how to continue, or to go on in the same way, after some instruction, even though, in principle, it might leave open a number of competing options. For that, in turn, to be the case, it might seem that some further intellectual process is needed to select just the right way to continue, perhaps an intuition, but as soon as one postulates a further inner guidance there will be a question of how it guides one (if an inner voice, how does it make itself known, in what language is it expressed, how should it be interpreted?).

Any further specification of the rule governing the series will have to face the fact that the student is supposed to learn how to apply that specification to new cases. That general moral applies even in the case of the banal series 2, 2, 2, 2 … The next digit has to be relevantly similar to what has gone before:

> But isn't *the same* at least the same? We seem to have an infallible paradigm of identity in the identity of a thing with itself. I feel like saying: 'Here at any rate there can't be a variety of interpretations. If you are seeing a thing you are seeing identity too.' Then are two things the same when they are what *one* thing is? And how am I to apply what the *one* thing shews me to the case of two things? (Wittgenstein 1953: §215)

Given the principled difficulty of determining the next step of a mathematical series and its open-ended nature, it is tempting to explain mastery of such series (by those who have mastered them) by ascribing a psychological mechanism that narrows down the range of future moves. As Wittgenstein shows, however, if inferring from finite past to future practice were not reliable in itself, postulating the intervening mechanism would not help either. Another person's past practice, once described as mere *inductive* evidence for a mechanism, could be evidence for any number of diverging mechanisms. Any finite number of examples might be interpreted to be in accord with an infinite number of possible continuations. It is easiest to think of this in the case of a third person ascription to another, but there are similar problems in the first person case, as well in ensuring that one embodies just the right mechanism oneself. If one specifies any actual causal mechanism to embody one's grasp of how the correct continuation must go, one is held hostage to the fortunes of that mechanism. Perhaps it will break down but, if so, that is not what one meant by 'add 2'. If instead one tries to specify an ideally functioning mechanism, then that merely replaces one symbolic form (representations of the series, or principles governing it from which later digits have to be derived) with another (an ideal description of a machine from which its movements have to be derived (cf. Wittgenstein 1953: §§193–4)).

Wittgenstein suggests that in both the first and third person cases, it is the apparent need for an *interpretation* that leads to a vicious regress. In the latter case, past practice has to be interpreted as following a particular rule. In the former, mental states, mental signs, processes or mechanisms have to be interpreted as determining a rule. Hence, Wittgenstein concludes:

> This was our paradox: no course of action could be determined by a rule, because every course of action can be made out to accord with the rule. The answer was: if everything can be made out to accord with the rule, then it can also be made out to conflict with it. And so there would be neither accord nor conflict here. It can be seen that there is a misunderstanding here from the mere fact that in the course of our argument we give one interpretation after another; as if each one contented us at least for a moment, until we thought of yet another standing behind it. What this shews is

that there is a way of grasping a rule which is *not* an *interpretation*, but which is exhibited in what we call 'obeying the rule' and 'going against it' in actual cases. (Wittgenstein 1953: §201)

The second half of the paragraph contains Wittgenstein's diagnosis of what gives rise to puzzlement about such learning and thus how to avoid it. Grasp of a rule does not consist in any mental phenomena coming before the mind's eye, which have to be interpreted to connect them to subsequent applications of the rule. Rather, understanding a rule is a basic practical ability, a piece of know-how. The attempt to explain such know-how through explicit knowledge falls foul of the regress of interpretations arguments. So, instead, it is know-how that is the more basic and this is accommodated in emphasis in the primacy of practice:

> Giving grounds, however, justifying the evidence, comes to an end;—but the end is not certain propositions' striking us immediately as true, i.e. it is not a kind of *seeing* on our part; it is our acting which lies at the bottom of the language game. (Wittgenstein 1969: §204)

Wittgenstein's discussion thus inverts the normal order of priority of explicit and tacit knowledge. Even in the case of judgements for which a universal principle can be written down, the ability to apply the principle depends on some basic shared practical responses to it. Justifications for those particular responses to a rule, however, come to an end. Fortunately, because humans share the same basic reactions, responses, routes of salience and so on, justifications typically come to an end in agreement. (If they did not, there would no such thing as shared linguistic or more generally conceptual order.) Thus, codified and uncodified judgements are, ultimately, in the same boat. Both depend on a tacit element.

Wittgenstein's discussion provides a powerful principled argument, which complements observations both about the role of experiment in clinical trials and about the application of such trials to specific cases, about the role of tacit knowledge in judgement. At the heart of explicit codified knowledge is judgement in accordance with rules, but whatever can be made explicit in specifying what does and what does not accord with a rule must itself inevitably rest on something implicit and tacit.

## A Wittgensteinian response to Hume's challenge to induction

Wittgenstein's discussion of rules also helps to shed light on Hume's account of the relation between justification of knowledge based on experience, and human custom and practice. Hume's challenge is to show how past experience can be taken to be a guide to the future without simply helping oneself to the claim that that is what has often been found to be the case in the past. To appeal to that, he suggests, is insufficient in itself without the further general principle that the past is a good guide to the future. This is either a premiss in a valid deductive argument, but one that would stand in need of further independent justification, or it is the principle of an inductive argument. If so, then the principle that was supposed to be justified (by appeal to its success in the past) has had to be presupposed (to show why what happened in the past is relevant) and thus the question has been begged. On either approach, there is a threat of a regress.

Wittgenstein's discussion of guidance by rules suggests a response to Hume's challenge to induction. Discussion of following a rule suggests that there is a similar challenge to deduction. Deduction depends on derivations that accord with rules, but as I have described, Wittgenstein presents a *prima facie* puzzle about how to justify the claim that a particular judgement is in accord with a general rule. Again, like Hume's challenge to induction, there is a threat of an infinite regress as soon as it seems necessary to encode, in a further higher rule, how the specification of a ground level rule is to be interpreted. The assumption that a judgement has always to be justified by subsuming it under a generalisation has to be rejected. Wittgenstein's positive suggestion, in this case, is that to understand a rule is just an ability to make applications of it without the need for further mediation by inner interpretations. Although there can be doubts about how to follow practical instruction, there need not be. One can be justified not by an infinite chain of higher level general rules, but by particular circumstances.

This Wittgensteinian lesson can also be applied to Hume's case as well. Whilst it may seem that a further inductive principle is needed to mediate between particular past experiences and judgements about the future, as soon as any such principle has to be consulted then a regress beckons. It beckons because the principle invoked also stands in need of a justification. How was it derived from experience? The regress can be blocked at the start by learning from Wittgenstein's discussion that judgements can be justified by particular circumstances. In Hume's case, judgements about the future can be justified by appealing to particular features of the past without also appealing to a further general rule.

As Hume himself pointed out, there is a custom or practice of making such judgements the practical necessity of which is not undermined by his own sceptical argument, but that fair point is not enough because it does not help defuse Humean scepticism about induction. A Wittgensteinian analysis of rule following adds three further related features, two of which have already been introduced.

First, Hume's challenge to induction implicitly compares induction unfavourably with deduction. Hume's own suggestion, that his deductive argument against induction showed that deduction, rather than induction, was at fault, is hard to take seriously. However, Wittgenstein's discussion suggests that deduction is, in one respect, in the same boat. Both are vulnerable to a threat of regress on the assumption that judgements need general justifications. So the aspect of the sceptical argument that depends on comparing induction unfavourably with deduction can be defused.

Secondly, as I have already described, the insight that enables Wittgensteinian scepticism to be blocked translates straight across to the Humean case. Humean scepticism gets off the ground through the assumption that judgements have to be justified through subsumption under more general rules, but that is a mistaken assumption.

A third feature should now also be clear. Hume's challenge works in part by calling for a defence of an approach to inductive practices from outside them. The justification should compel even someone with no mastery of inductive judgements. With that restriction in place, the challenge is impossible to meet. The parallel challenge to deductive practices and rule following more generally also calls for a defence from outside shared reactions and again, so set up, the challenge is impossible to meet, but the felt need to justify our practices from a position of 'cosmic exile' is spurious (Quine 1960: 275). In both cases, the attempt to step outside human practices and justify them from outside is doomed to fail.

This is not to say that epistemic practices should not be scrutinised and questioned, but such scrutiny has to take some things for granted to start with. Examining both Hume and Wittgenstein shows that this is a fundamental feature of rational judgement, rather than a sign of sloppy thinking. The attempt to justify knowledge claims by appeal to higher level principles cannot escape the fact that such principles themselves depend on particular judgements in the face of particular facts.

## 5. Conclusions

Evidence-based medicine concerns how best to learn from experience. It contains specific concrete advice summarised in the evidence hierarchy. In the hierarchy, more general methods are ranked above less general. Thus, meta-analysis is higher than single randomised control trials, which are ranked higher than non-experimental, descriptive studies, which are higher than individual clinical judgement. The ranking makes a claim about what forms of evidence are better, in the sense of increasing the chances that clinical judgement is true and thus treatment and management will be successful. What, then, underpins that claim? Is it, itself, based on evidence? Or does it follow from *a priori*, philo-sophical reasoning?

To take the second option first: some *a priori* arguments can be given in support of the ranking. It seems, in principle, that forms of evidence higher up the list will be less vulnerable to particular kinds of bias than those lower down the list. Randomisation, for example, helps eliminate an uncontrolled-for factor influencing an investigation of a target causal factor. At heart, the method of clinical trails against a control underpins much of EBM and is based on Mill's method of difference. It does seem to be a method underpinned by *a priori* analysis. The method follows from the meanings of 'necessity' and 'sufficiency' as a way of eliminating conditions that cannot be necessary or sufficient for an effect. (Although this chapter has not discussed the analysis of causation, there is a *prima facie* connection between it and those strictly logical notions.) However, as is clear on reflection, the method of difference (like the method of agreement) cannot strictly be applied in practice. It is not possible to meet the initial conditions specified. Thus whilst some arguments can be given for why ascending the hierarchy tends to eliminate sources of bias, it is very unlikely that the hierarchy can be given purely *a priori* or philosophical defence.

What then of the first option? Can substantive claims about what forms of evidence are most reliable itself be based on evidence? The answer to this is a qualified 'yes'. Evidence can be brought to bear, but not unquestionable evidence. One might, for example, compare the effectiveness of mental health care, rates of recovery and so forth, before and after the rise of EBM. But counting such a descriptive study as providing positive evidence for EBM (on the assumption that it does) presupposes that that form of evidence is reliable. Consider now the possibility of conflicting results from different kinds of study, large descriptive studies, small-scale experimental studies and so on. Only if one has already ranked the forms of evidence will one know how to assess the conflicting results, but such ranking is just what was supposed to be under investigation.

This suggests that taking EBM seriously involves recognising that its prescriptions are themselves scientific claims about the world and stand in need of critical reflection no less than does any particular empirical trial of particular treatments in mental health. As careful consideration of Hume's challenge to induction suggests, such reflection has itself to stand within a tradition. It is impossible to step outside our epistemic practices and justify them from scratch.

Defusing Humean scepticism does not, of course, remove all difficulties from assessing inductive evidence. A number of everyday empirical problems remain which include assessing the representativeness of samples, the extent to which confounding causal factors are controlled for and other difficulties created through the only partial application of Mill's method of difference to actual situations. These are, however, best dealt with through a balance of formal procedures and clinical judgement.

Returning to the account of EBM in psychiatry discussed at the start of the chapter, in fairness, Geddes and Harrison emphasise some of the complexities in the process of applying the results of clinical trails in practical clinical contexts. Thus, although they argue that, ideally, treatment options should be based on evidence of effectiveness from a source as high up the list of favoured forms of evidence as possible, they also point out that the evidence of clinical trials has also to be *relevant* to the case at hand. So a further assessment has to be made of whether the subjects involved in the trial are a close enough match for the actual patient. Subjects in trials may be all of the same sex and they may be less likely to have only a single medical condition. What should also be pointed out is that complexities do not simply affect the practical application of such clinical findings, but also the scientific process of arriving at findings in the first place.

Thus, a proper understanding of EBM plays up, rather than playing down the need for critical judgement in assessing evidence. Here, there is a key role for the subjects engaged in scientific psychiatry to exercise skilled judgement in a way that is only ever partly codifiable.

# Conclusions and the future of philosophy of psychiatry

The six chapters of this book have offered a snapshot of the diverse subjects that make up contemporary philosophy of psychiatry, but whilst they have ranged across the three main themes of the role of values, understanding meanings and the scientific and factual basis of mental health care, there have been some underlying common conclusions that have been re-emphasised throughout the book.

In this brief final section, I will highlight three such unifying conclusions:

◆ there is an ineliminable role for non-algorithmic or uncodified judgement in mental health care;

◆ the basic unit of meaning or significance is the whole person;

◆ the best understanding of nature is a relaxed rather than a reductionist naturalism.

## The role of judgement

Throughout the book I have emphasised the important role that judgement, as in the phase 'having good judgement', has to play in mental health care. This notion stands in opposition to codified or algorithmic practice. Thus, it is worth reflecting on the increasing emphasis that has been placed on codification of psychiatric practice.

One reason for the increasing emphasis on codification is the focus on reliability of diagnosis in medicine in general and psychiatry in particular. This has been most obvious in the emphasis on operationalism in psychiatric diagnosis since DSM-III, but it is also shown in the rise of structured and semi-structured interview protocols originating, within psychiatry, with the Present State Examination. Codifications of diagnosis or of interview techniques promise to standardise clinical judgements, and thus improve communication between clinicians and research.

Such codifications are also present outside diagnosis, however. They are present in the emphasis, in the UK at least, on the management of risk, rather than diagnosis or therapy. Risk management is increasingly governed by algorithmic procedures, rather than clinical judgement. Yet more broadly, in the

UK, the General Medical Council publishes substantial ethical guidelines in *Good Medical Practice*, for example. Medical school syllabuses are substantially defined in *Tomorrow's Doctors* and so forth. There is also, of course, a background of relevant medical law.

In general, codifications have a number of practical purposes. As well as facilitating communication and research for doctors, they can help define minimum standards of care for service users and set out an agreed legal framework against which judgements of permissible actions can be made.

There is, however, also a danger of thinking that codifications can do something more then just partially specify minimum standards of care. It might be thought that they can capture the nature of skilled clinical judgement itself. This assumption can be backed up by the following intuitive argument. *Contrary to anti-psychiatric criticisms, psychiatry does succeed at least partially in classifying, diagnosing and managing the medical conditions of service users. This involves making judgements about objective matters, judgements that can be right or wrong. However, to be such an objective judgement requires a standard of rightness and wrongness and that in turn requires a codification.*

Against such a background argument, denying that judgements of facts, values and meanings can, in general, be codified can seem like a form of anti-psychiatry, but it is not. Nor does it encourage a shallow form of relativism of the 'anything goes' variety. Rather the idea is that the assumption that judgements are algorithmic should be replaced by the idea that they are responsive to clinical contexts in a way that is not easily predictable. A skilled practitioner is able to make judgements that aim to get situations right. In mental health care, this involves a complex inter-relation between factual, meaningful and evaluative aspects. Within each of these aspects, judgements will depend on the relations between different reasons pulling in different ways. Thus, the overall judgement is based on an appreciation of a complex whole, but this is not to say that the interaction of the factors that make up the whole can be predicted algorithmically.

Appreciating that psychiatric judgement resists codification has a practical consequence. The unrealistic emphasis on the possibility of codification risks:

- abusive practice, when values are squeezed into a constraining framework;
- misunderstanding, when meanings are treated mechanically;
- less than optimally evidence-based practice, when the element of judgement about the relevance of evidence is downplayed.

To see the proper significance of objective but uncodified judgement in all three key aspects of psychiatry is to free psychiatric practice from a dangerous distorting influence.

# The basic unit of meaning is the whole person

In Chapter 4, I contrasted cognitivism with a constructionist version of discursive psychology. Although quite different in emphasis, both are attempts to reduce facts about the meaning of utterances and the content of mental states to something more basic. The reductionist ambition is clearer in the case of cognitivist approaches to psychiatry, which aim to describe mental states in information processing terms. Whilst this is not always spelled out, the meaning of utterances is supposed to be based on the content of mental states and these in turn are explained through the information carried by internal states—or representations—processed in the brain or nervous system. This leaves the question of how individual mental representations are injected with meaning or content, with either causal theories or evolutionary theories being the favoured attempted solutions in philosophy.

Constructionist discursive approaches, on the other hand, invert the priority of explanation. The content of mental states is explained as constructed in public utterances. This is, again, reductionist, and both radical and revisionary because there is no room for the idea that an utterance might answer to and accurately express a prior mental state.

Drawing on arguments from Wittgenstein, however, I argued that neither approach is right because neither can capture the normativity implicit in both meaning and content. Meaning cannot be reduced to more basic non-normative phenomena or processes. Instead, it comes into view only at a level of description of whole persons, rather than either states of the brain or nervous system or autonomous linguistic codes. The basic unit of meaning is thus a living, whole person.

However, whilst that claim applies most clearly to the discussion of Chapter 4, it is helpful in a number of other places. Thus, for example, it helps to contextualise the development of a model of comprehensive diagnosis, with a narrative formulation tailored to individual subjects, which was discussed in Chapter 5. Such diagnosis aims to get right the nature of the whole person because that is the level at which experiences can be understood to have meaning or significance.

It also complements the criticism, in Chapter 2, of the idea that moral or ethical judgements might be codified in both contentful and consistent principles. Rejecting principlism, I argued for a form of moral particularism. Now, however, the idea that the basic unit of meaning is a person helps put into context the 'object' of particular moral judgements. Such judgements turn on the interaction of real people, rather than the mathematical addition of ethical principles.

The role of uncodified judgement and the importance of persons as the basic level at which meaning comes into view are thus two ideas that complement one another. These are not put forward, however, for political or aesthetic reasons relating to how I think mental health care should be practiced. Rather, they follow from analysis of the very idea of judgement and meaning.

## Relaxed naturalism

The third element is perhaps the most clearly philosophical. It has to do with the nature of nature. One widespread aspect of contemporary thought is that nature is exhausted by the description that will eventually be offered by a completed physics. In a book on meaning, the assumption that all natural phenomena are really physical is shaped into an explicit argument by the philosopher Jerry Fodor, which is worth quoting at length:

> I suppose that sooner or later the physicists will complete the catalogue they've been compiling of the ultimate and irreducible properties of things. When they do, the likes of *spin*, *charm* and *charge* will perhaps appear upon their list. But *aboutness* surely won't; intentionality simply doesn't go that deep. It's hard to see, in face of this consideration, how one can be a Realist about intentionality without also being, to some extent or other, a Reductionist. If the semantic and intentional are real properties of things, it must be in virtue of their identity with (or maybe of their supervenience on?) properties that are *neither* intentional *nor* semantic. If aboutness is real, it must be really something else. (Fodor 1987: 97)

Fodor's argument takes it for granted that a complete catalogue of physical properties is a complete catalogue of nature. With this assumption in place, a necessary condition for a property to be a genuine or real feature of the world is either that it is found in that catalogue of physical properties or that it can, at least, be related to properties found there. If, by contrast, no such relation obtains then the problematic concepts cannot describe genuine features of the world.

This meta-*physical* view gives rise to a characteristic meta-*philosophical* view. Philosophy should aim to 'naturalise' problematic concepts, ideas or phenomena by relating them back to the more basic vocabulary of natural science or physics that serves as a standard or benchmark. Showing how a philosophically puzzling phenomenon can be reduced to (or constructed from) something more basic and not puzzling should ease philosophical confusion. Naturalism so understood is a form of reductionism.

The idea that a physical description of the world can serve as a benchmark for what is real is applied in a number of different areas. In the quotation from Fodor, the idea is applied to the nature of meaning, but it also underpins reductionist accounts of mental illness discussed in Chapter 1 and the neo-Humean approaches to ethics described in Chapters 2 and 5. These assume that ethical judgements have to be understood as projections of sentiments onto a value-free physical world, rather than as responses to genuine moral facts.

I have argued, however, that reductionist analyses of mental illness, moral judgement and understanding meaning face grave difficulties. If they are, as I have argued, false hopes, what then of the nature of nature?

The suggestion that I have set out in the book is derived from the philosopher John McDowell's explicit consideration of the significance of any failure in philosophy to reduce complex concepts such as moral value or meaning to more basic ones. Rather than regarding such failure as impugning the reality or worldliness of the properties or concepts concerned, it may merely show that reductionists have started with an impoverished conception of what is real or part of nature. McDowell suggests that, although the assumption that what is real is exhausted by the natural sciences is itself a natural one it is by no means compulsory:

> What is at work here is a conception of nature that can seem sheer common sense, though it was not always so; the conception I mean was made available only by a hard-won achievement of human thought at a specific time, the time of the rise of modern science. Modern science understands its subject matter in a way that threatens, at least, to leave it disenchanted. (McDowell 1994: 70)

One reason for saying that science leaves its subject matter 'disenchanted' is that the mediaeval idea that nature comprised a book of moral lessons has been rightly rejected, but in addition McDowell suggests that it threatens to limit what is real to what he calls the 'realm of law'. This contrasts with those phenomena that have to be fitted within a different pattern of intelligibility: the 'space of reasons' (in Sellars' phrase) that describes the rational pattern of intentional states. He suggests that nature should not be equated just with the realm of law, but should also be taken to include the space of reasons.

By suggesting that nature includes more than just what lies within the realm of law, McDowell does not aim to slight the success of science. Nor does he suggest that there should be no place for a disenchanted view of nature within scientific method:

> But it is one thing to recognise that the impersonal stance of scientific investigation is a methodological necessity for the achievement of a valuable mode of understanding reality; it is quite another thing to take the dawning grasp of this, in the modern era, for a metaphysical insight into the notion of objectivity as such, so that objective correctness in any mode of thought must be anchored in this kind of access to the real … [It] is not the educated common sense it represents itself as being; it is shallow metaphysics. (McDowell 1998b: 182)

The moral that McDowell draws and that I have hinted at in this book is that there is more to nature than can be described within the natural sciences.

Nature is broader than that. This is not to advance an anti-scientific claim. Science has been very successful in explaining a range of phenomena by subsuming them under general laws, but that need not imply that phenomena that cannot be so set out are not real.

In the context of this book, this anti-reductionist or relaxed version of naturalism suggests that the wider concerns of mental health care can be accommodated within a broader conception of what is really real. In addition to the hard bio-medical facts, the demands of both values and meanings can be seen to be real features of the world and thus real features of the clinical situation calling for skilled judgement.

## The future of philosophy of psychiatry

If the diverse areas addressed by the six chapters of this book represent some of the main themes making up the present state of philosophy of psychiatry, what of its future?

One possibility is that the diversity of the new philosophy of psychiatry is a temporary phenomenon. It might be, in Kuhnian terms, an aspect of the revolutionary birth (or rebirth) of the subject within broader analytic or Anglo-American philosophy. If so, one might expect it to evolve into its normal science phase, characterised by an agreed agenda of puzzles to be worked through within an agreed methodological framework. It might become more like the philosophy of mind or epistemology with a settled role within the philosophical canon.

I do not believe, however, that the subject will or should evolve like this. Philosophy of psychiatry or, more broadly, philosophy of mental health care is primarily a philosophy of and for mental health care. It is at its best when it responds to questions and examines the conceptual underpinning of developing thought in this area. This, in turn, makes prediction of the future of philosophy of psychiatry difficult.

It is reasonable, however, to expect that future developments in philosophy of psychiatry will be based, in part, on current developments both in philosophy and, in the broader context, of mental health care. I will outline just three.

In the philosophy of mind, there has been a rise in influence of accounts of the mind that start with the embedded, embodied, and *enactive nature* of human subjects or agents. This contrasts with those views, described in Chapter 4, which approach the mind as an information processing computer, processing internal representations of the outer world. Enactivist accounts of the mind were presented at a recent International Conference on Philosophy Psychiatry and Psychology in Leiden in 2006 and used, for example, to attempt to interpret brain imaging experiments.

I predict that there will be further work in philosophy of mind in exploring the connections between enactivism and broadly consistent approaches, such as Wittgensteinian and neo-Fregean approaches within analytic philosophy and phenomenological approaches informed by Heidegger and Merleau-Ponty within continental philosophy. However, this work will also be more widely applied to psychopathology in both careful descriptions and potential explanations of subjects' experiences.

There has been a recent revival within moral philosophy of *virtue ethics*, which places moral character at the heart of ethical thinking, contrasting with principles-based approaches, whether deontological or consequentialist. A similar view has also spread to epistemology under the title 'virtue epistemology'. The analysis of knowledge starts not with the nature and pedigree of beliefs, but rather with an analysis of the virtues manifested by knowing subjects. It is thus person based.

I predict that just as virtue ethics have begun to be applied within medicine, as a reaction to conventional principles-based medical ethics, so virtue epistemology will be used to examine the nature of clinical expertise as a reaction against the shortcomings of the overemphasis on codification by evidence-based medicine.

From the *clinical* side, there are a number of developing themes that are interrelated. These include:

◆ the rise of a human rights approach to mental health contrasted with public fears of risk;

◆ the growth of what is called a 'recovery model', in contrast to a medical model;

◆ the idea of citizenship and the role of subjects as members of communities as important resources for better understanding mental health care.

Whilst these ideas have all been discussed they have yet to be given a fully-integrated in-depth philosophical treatment. Thus, for example, the recovery model has been widely debated, but no model has yet been articulated that really does contest or rival a medical model (which is itself, despite its wide-spread currency, far from fully developed as a *model* of healthcare). I expect both further analysis of the 'logical geography' of these concepts, and the articulation of philosophically robust models and analyses to contribute to, and inform, public debate about the future of mental health care.

Whatever precise future developments there are, what should be clear is the need for and the rude health of the philosophy of psychiatry.

# Philosophical glossary

*a posteriori*: an epistemological term meaning capable of being known only with experience. The contrast is *a priori*.

*a priori*: an epistemological term meaning capable of being known prior to or independently of experience. The contrast is *a posteriori*.

**analytic**: a semantic term meaning true in virtue of meaning alone. The contrast is synthetic.

**behaviourism**: in philosophy of mind, the view that mental states are behavioural dispositions.

**biological function**: although there are competing accounts of functions, roughly speaking, a biological system has a function if the behaviour of the system best explains its continued existence, via past evolutionary success. Functions are normative and, thus, might be used to explain both the content of mental states and the nature of illness, disease or disorder.

**causal theory of reference**: within the philosophy of thought and language the name for an approach that explains the content of mental states as whatever causes them.

*ceteris paribus*: literally 'all other things being equal'. It is used to qualify the laws of special sciences, such as social sciences, which only apply if background conditions are met. The contrasting case would be a set of laws, perhaps in basic physics, which applied universally.

**cognitivism**: in philosophy of psychiatry, the view that mental states are inner states of an information processing system. It is closely related to representationalism in philosophy of thought and language, and to functionalism in the philosophy of mind.

**consequentialism**: the view that the moral value of an ethical judgement or action depends only on whether it has good consequences. The most famous example of consequentialism is Mill's Utilitarianism.

**constitutive principle of rationality**: the claim, associated with Donald Davidson, that rationality plays a constitutive role for mental states. Rationality thus distinguishes the space of reasons from the realm of law.

**constructionism**: in philosophy of thought and language, the claim that phenomena such as mental states or meanings are constructed in ongoing social interaction. Discursive psychology is usually taken to be constructionist.

**constructive empiricism**: a view in the philosophy of science associated with Van Fraassen that science should aim merely at 'saving the phenomena' or producing correct observational predictions, whilst remaining agnostic about the truth of the implications it has for unobservable phenomena. The contrast is with a form of realism.

**contingent**: a metaphysical term used to characterise those truths that might have been otherwise. This is sometimes expressed by saying that they are true in only some possible worlds. The contrast is one sense of necessity.

**deontology**: the view that the moral value of an action is independent of the action's actual consequences, but depends instead on one or more general duties to act.

**discursive psychology**: an approach within the philosophy of psychiatry that views mental states as essentially public and tied to linguistic utterances. The main contrast is cognitivism.

**disease entity assumption**: the assumption that diagnostic categories are valid and thus reflect real and causally active disease entities.

**epistemology**: the study of knowledge, the 'logos' of knowledge.

**estranged epistemology**: an account of knowledge of the world, or intentionality more broadly, which assumes that subjects have access to the world only via scrutiny of internal representations of it. It contrasts with more practical approaches.

**explanation**: in addition to its everyday meaning, in the philosophy of the social sciences it carries an implicit connection to explanation of phenomena by subsuming them under general laws. The contrast is understanding.

*eudaemonia*: a Greek word often translated as happiness, but best understood more broadly to mean flourishing.

**falsificationism**: a view in the philosophy of science associated with Popper that science should aim to reject false theories through conjecture and refutation, rather than aim to provide positive support. It is a response to the problem of justifying induction.

**functionalism**: in the philosophy of mind, the view that mental states are characterised in terms of their causal inputs and outputs. On this view, the mind stands to the brain as software to hardware. It is related to representationalism in the philosophy of thought and language, and cognitivism in philosophy of psychiatry.

**genetic understanding**: according to Jaspers, a form of empathic understanding of the way one mental state arises, ideally and typically, from another. The contrast is, more generally, with explanation by subsumption under natural laws and, more specifically, with static understanding.

**idiographic**: a term deployed by Windelband to mean an understanding of individual cases according to their unique and individual aspects. The contrast is nomothetic.

**induction**: this normally means reasoning from particular cases to generalities. Such reasoning is, more precisely, called 'enumerative induction' and attempting to justify it in general is called the 'problem of induction', highlighted by Hume. Mill uses 'eliminative induction' to describe his ideal experimental methods of isolating necessary and sufficient conditions.

**intentionality**: the capacity of mental states and linguistic utterances to be about things, to refer and to be true or false.

**likeness argument**: the name for an argument to establish the status of mental illness. It either takes a paradigmatic form of physical illness and shows that mental illness is sufficiently like it because it shares sufficient of its features, or it abstracts a generic concept of illness (typically from physical illness) and shows that mental illness fits sufficient features of that general concept to count as illness.

**master thesis**: the thesis that mental states are not essentially relational states and have, instead, to be connected to aspects of the world by interpretations. McDowell suggests that the master thesis is both a key component of the Cartesian picture of mind and also the key target of Wittgenstein's rule following considerations.

**metaphysics**: literally 'after nature' meaning the book that followed the book on nature (called 'physics') in Aristotle's works. It now refers to a very general and high level investigation of reality including the preconditions for empirical investigation of nature, and the fundamental concepts used in that investigation. It is thus related to, but broader than, ontology.

**myth of the given**: the name given by Sellars for a version of epistemological foundationalism based on the idea that there are foundational beliefs that are non-inferentially arrived at, presuppose no other beliefs and constitute the ultimate court of appeal for factual claims.

**naturalism:** the name of an approach to philosophy with the aim of understanding how puzzling phenomena, such as meanings or values, can be fitted into an unproblematic understanding of nature. The most common form is reductionist naturalism, which aims to explain puzzling concepts in more basic terms.

**necessary**: this term has two meanings in philosophy. In its metaphysical sense it means 'not possibly not' and refers to truths that could not have been otherwise. They are true in all possible worlds. The contrast is with contingent. In logic it means 'without which not' and refers to conditions that have to obtain for some further condition to obtain. The contrast is with sufficient because if A is sufficient for B then B is necessary for A.

**nomological**: governed by natural laws.

**nomothetic**: a term deployed by Windelband to mean an understanding of individual or general phenomena in general terms via subsumption under general laws. The contrast is idiographic.

**normativity**: in the philosophy of thought and language, the prescriptive quality of mental states and linguistic utterances exemplified in what makes a belief true or false or what satisfies or frustrates a hope or intention. In philosophy of psychiatry, it may apply to the good or bad aspect of health and illness.

**ontology**: the study of what exists, the 'logos' of being.

**particularism**: in moral philosophy, the view that ethical judgements cannot be codified in principles and, instead, answer to particular value-laden worldly situations. The contrast is principlism.

**positivists**: the name for philosophers who espouse a scientific model of philosophy and stress the importance of what can be measured and detected. The Logical Positivists were a group based around the Vienna Circle of the 1930s who promoted the Verification Principle which states that meaning of a sentence is its method of verification.

**principlism**: in moral philosophy, the view that ethical judgements can be codified in principles. A central example is deontology.

**qualia**: the qualitative aspects of mental phenomena, the felt quality of experiences when, for example, looking at a colour or tasting something.

**realm of law**: a phrase popularised by McDowell to refer to those phenomena that can be explained by subsumption under natural laws.

***reductio ad absurdum***: a form of logical argument in which a contradiction is derived from a set of premises implying that at least one premiss must be false.

**reductionism**: the attempt to explain complex and puzzling phenomena in more basic terms. Reductionism is usually carried out against a background assumption that a completed basic physical science provides the benchmark for what is real and, thus, what is neither within a completed basic physics nor reducible to it, is not real.

**representationalism**: in the philosophy of thought and language, the view that mental states are encoded in inner neurological states that represent features of the outer world. It is often combined with a causal theory of reference or teleosemantics.

**semantics:** the aspects of a language and by extension thought that have to do with truth and reference. It is connected to intentionality. One contrast is with the syntax of a language.

**simulation theory:** the view in the philosophy of mind that our knowledge of other minds is based not on having an implicit theory of mind, but simply having a mind and imaginatively putting oneself in the position of others. The usual contrast is theory theory.

**space of reasons:** a metaphorical name for the rational structure of beliefs and concepts popularised by McDowell who explicitly mentions relations of implication and probability as examples of the relations that structure the space. The contrast is with the realm of law.

**stance stance:** a philosophical approach which aims to shed light on puzzling phenomena by examining the interpretative stance used to describe or make sense of them.

**static understanding:** according to Jaspers, a form of empathic understanding of the nature and quality of kinds of mental state. Jaspers also calls this 'phenomenology'. The contrast is more generally with explanation by subsumption under natural laws and, more specifically, with genetic understanding.

**sufficient:** a condition is sufficient for another if it guarantees that the second condition obtains. The contrast is necessity: if A is sufficient for B then B is necessary for A.

**supervenience:** a notion originally developed by Moore to apply to the relation between ethical and non-ethical worldly properties, but now more usually used to characterise the relation of mind and body. Mental properties supervene on physical properties if and only if a change of mental properties implies a change of physical properties, but a change of physical properties need not imply a change of mental properties (because, for example, mental states can be realised in more than one way, physically).

**synthetic:** a semantic term meaning true in virtue both of meaning and also a worldly feature together. The contrast is analytic.

**teleosemantics:** the approach in the philosophy of thought and language to explain or naturalise meaning, broadly construed, through evolutionary theory. The main idea is that a mental state has the meaning or content that it has a biological function to carry.

**theory theory:** the view in the philosophy of mind that our knowledge of other minds is based on knowledge of an implicit theory of how mental states are related to perceptual inputs and behavioural outputs. It is related to functionalism as the epistemological correlative of that ontological account of the nature of mental states. The usual contrast is simulation theory.

**understanding:** in addition to its everyday meaning, in the philosophy of the social sciences it carries an implicit connection to understanding phenomena through charting their meaning. Jaspers distinguishes between static and genetic understanding. The contrast is explanation.

**virtue ethics:** the view that the moral value of ethical judgement depends on the character of a moral subject.

# Bibliography

American Psychiatric Association (1952) *Diagnostic and Statistical Manual of Mental Disorders First Edition (DSM-I)*. Washington, DC: American Psychiatric Association.

American Psychiatric Association (1968) *Diagnostic and Statistical Manual of Mental Disorders Second Edition (DSM-II)*. Washington, DC: American Psychiatric Association.

American Psychiatric Association (1980) *Diagnostic and Statistical Manual of Mental Disorders Third Edition (DSM-III)*. Washington, DC: American Psychiatric Association.

American Psychiatric Association (1987) *Diagnostic and Statistical Manual of Mental Disorders Third Edition Revised (DSM-III-R)*. Washington, DC: American Psychiatric Association.

American Psychiatric Association (1994) *Diagnostic and Statistical Manual of Mental Disorders Fourth Edition (DSM-IV)*. Washington, DC: American Psychiatric Association.

Anastasi, A. (1968) *Psychological testing*. New York: Macmillan.

Aristotle (2000) *Nicomachean Ethics*. Cambridge: Cambridge University Press.

Austin, J.L. (1957) A plea for excuses. *Proceedings of the Aristotelian Society* 57: 1–30.

Austin, J.L. (1962) *Sense and Sensibilia*. Oxford: Oxford University Press.

Bayer, R. and Spitzer, R.L. (1985) Neurosis, psychodynamics and DSM-III. *Archives of General Psychiatry* 42: 187–96.

Beauchamp, T.L. (2003) Methods and principles in biomedical ethics. *Journal of Medical Ethics* 29: 269–274.

Beauchamp, T.L. and Childress, J.F. (2001) *Principles of Biomedical Ethics*. Oxford: Oxford University Press.

Bedau, M. (1998) Where's the good in teleology? In: Allen, C. and Lauder, G. (Eds) *Nature's Purposes: analyses of function and design in biology*. Cambridge: MIT Press, 261–91.

Berrios, G. (1991) Delusions as 'wrong beliefs': a conceptual history. *British Journal of Psychiatry* 159 (suppl 14): 6–13.

Blackburn, S. (1984) *Spreading the Word*. Oxford: Oxford University Press.

Blackburn, S. (2000) *Ruling Passions*. Oxford: Oxford University Press.

Bolton, D. and Hill, J. (2004) *Mind, Meaning and Mental Disorder*. Oxford: Oxford University Press.

Boorse, C. (1975) On the distinction between disease and illness. *Philosophy and Public Affairs* 5: 49–68.

Boorse, C. (1998) What a theory of mental health should be. In: Green, S.A. and Bloch, S. (Eds) *An Anthology of Psychiatric Ethics*. Oxford: Oxford University Press, 108–15.

Boyd, R. (1999) On the current status of scientific realism. In: Boyd, R., Gasker, P. and Trout, J.D. (Eds) *The Philosophy of Science*. Cambridge: MIT Press, 195–222.

Brandom, R. (1994) *Making it Explicit*. Cambridge: Harvard University Press.

Bridgman, P.W. (1927) *The Logic of Modern Physics*. New York: Macmillan.

Campbell, J. (2001) Rationality, meaning and the analysis of delusion. In: *Philosophy Psychiatry and Psychology* 8: 89–100.

Cartwright, N. (1983) *How the Laws of Physics Lie*. Oxford: Oxford University Press.

Cartwright, N. (1999) *The Dappled World: a study of the boundaries of science.* Cambridge: Cambridge University Press.

Cavell, S. (1969) The availability of Wittgenstein's later philosophy. In: *Must We Mean What We Say?* Cambridge: Cambridge University Press, 44–72.

Chodoff, P. (1984) Involuntary hospitalisation of the mentally ill as a moral issue. *American Journal of Psychiatry* 141: 384–9.

Collins, H. (1985) *Changing Order: replication and induction in scientific practice.* London: Sage.

Cooper, R. (2002) Disease. *Studies in History and Philosophy of Biological and Biomedical Sciences* 33: 263–82.

Cooper, R. (2004) What is wrong with the DSM? *History of Psychiatry* 15: 5–25.

Corner, L. and Bond, J. (2006) The impact of the label of Mild Cognitive Impairment on the individual's sense of self. *Philosophy, Psychiatry and Psychology* 13: 3–12.

Crary, A. and Read, R. (2000) *The New Wittgenstein.* London: Routledge.

Dancy, J. (1993) *Moral Reasons.* Oxford: Blackwell.

Davidson, D. (1980) *Essays on Actions and Events.* Oxford: Oxford University Press.

Davidson, D. (1984) *Inquiries into Truth and Interpretation.* Oxford: Oxford University Press.

Davies, M., Coltheart, M., Langdon, R. and Breen, N. (2002) Monothematic delusions: towards a two-factor account. *Philosophy, Psychiatry and Psychology* 9: 133–58.

Dennett, D. (1987) *The Intentional Stance.* Cambridge: MIT Press.

Dretske, F.I. (1981) *Knowledge and the Flow of Information.* Oxford: Blackwell.

Edwards, D. and Potter, J. (1992) *Discursive Psychology.* London: Sage.

Ehrlich, E., Ehrlich, L. and Pepper, G.B. (Eds) (1986) *Karl Jaspers: basic philosophical writings.* Athens: Ohio University Press.

Eilan, N. (2000) On understanding schizophrenia. In: Zahavi, D. (Ed.) *Exploring the self.* Amsterdam: John Benjamins, 97–113.

Ellis, A.W. (1996) *Human Cognitive Neuropsychology: a textbook with readings.* Hove: Psychology Press.

Elstein, A.S., Shulman, L.S. and Sprafka, S.A. (1978) *Medical Problem Solving: an analysis of clinical reasoning.* Cambridge: Harvard University Press.

Fine, A. (1986) The natural ontological attitude. In: *The Shaky Game.* Chicago: University of Chicago Press, 112–35.

Fodor, J. (1975) *The Language of Thought.* Hassocks: Harvester.

Fodor, J. (1987) *Psychosemantics: the problem of meaning in the philosophy of mind.* Cambridge: MIT Press.

Fodor, J. and Chihara, C. (1965) Operationalism and ordinary language: a critique of Wittgenstein. *American Philosophical Quarterly* 2: 281–95.

Freud, S. (2002) *The Psychopathology of Everyday Life.* London: Penguin.

Frith, C. (1992) *The Cognitive Neuropsychology of Schizophrenia.* Hove: Lawrence Erlbaum.

Fulford, K.W.M. (1989) *Moral Theory and Medical Practice.* Cambridge: Cambridge University Press.

Fulford, K.W.M. (1991) The concept of disease. In: Bloch, S. and Chodoff, P. (Eds) *Psychiatric Ethics* (2nd edn). Oxford: Oxford University Press, 77–99.

Fulford, K.W.M. (1999a) Analytic philosophy, brain science and the concept of disorder. In: Bloch, S. Chodoff, P. and Green, S.A. (Eds) *Psychiatric Ethics* (3rd edn). Oxford: Oxford University Press, 161–92.

Fulford, K.W.M. (1999b) Nine variations and a coda on the theme of an evolutionary definition of dysfunction. *Journal of Abnormal Psychology* 108: 412–20.

Fulford, K.W.M. (2000) Teleology without tears. *Philosophy, Psychiatry and Psychology* 7: 77–94.

Fulford, K.W.M. (2004) Ten principles of values-based medicine. In: Radden, J. (ed) *The Philosophy of Psychiatry: a companion*. New York: Oxford University Press, 205–34.

Fulford, K.W.M. and Hope, T. (1993) Psychiatric ethics: a bioethical ugly duckling? In: Gillon, R. and Lloyd, A. (Eds) *Principles of Health Care Ethics*. New York: John Wiley and Sons Ltd, 681–95.

Fulford, K.W.M., Thornton, T. and Graham, G. (2006) *Oxford Textbook of Philosophy and Psychiatry*. Oxford: Oxford University Press.

Galtung, J. (1969) *Theory and Methods of Social Research*. Oslo: Universitetsforlaget.

Geddes, J.R. and Harrison, P.J. (1997) Closing the gap between research and practice. *British Journal of Psychiatry* 171: 220–5.

Gillon, R. (2003) Ethics needs principles—four can encompass the rest—and respect for autonomy should be 'first among equals'. *Journal of Medical Ethics* 29: 307–12.

Gipps, R.G.T. and Fulford, K.W.M. (2004) Understanding the clinical concept of delusion: from an estranged to an engaged epistemology. *International Review of Psychiatry* 16: 225–35.

Goodman, N. (1983) *Fact, Fiction and Forecast*. Harvard: Harvard University Press.

Harari, E. (2001) Whose evidence? Lessons from the philosophy of science and the epistemology of medicine. *Australian and New Zealand Journal of Psychiatry* 35: 724–30.

Hare, R.M. (1952) *The Language of Morals*. Oxford: Oxford University Press.

Hare, R.M. (1967) The promising game. In: Foot, P. (Ed.) *Theories of Ethics*. Oxford: Oxford University Press, 115–27.

Harre, R. and Gillett, G. (1994) *The Discursive Mind*. London: Sage.

Heal, J. (1995) Replication and functionalism. In: Davies, M. and Stone, T. (Eds) *Folk Psychology*. Oxford: Blackwell, 45–59.

Heidegger, M. (1962) *Being and Time*. Oxford: Blackwell.

Hempel, C.G. (1994) Fundamentals of taxonomy. In: Sadler, J.S. Wiggins, O.P. and Schwartz, M.A. (Eds) *Philosophical Perspectives on Psychiatric Diagnostic Classification*. Baltimore: Johns Hopkins University Press, 315–31.

Hosking, D.M. and Morley, I.E. (2004) Editorial: special issue on social constructionist praxis. *Journal of Community and Applied Psychology* 14: 318–31.

Hume, D. ([1748] 1975) *Enquiries Concerning the Human Understanding and Concerning the Principles of Morals*. Oxford: Clarendon Press.

Hurley, S. (1998) *Consciousness in Action*. Cambridge: Harvard University Press.

Jaspers, K. ([1912] 1968) The phenomenological approach in psychopathology. *British Journal of Psychiatry* 114: 1313–23.

Jaspers, K. ([1913] 1974) Causal and 'meaningful' connections between life history and psychosis, transl. by Hoenig J. In: Hirsch, S.R. and Shepherd, M. (Eds) *Themes and Variations in European Psychiatry*. Bristol: Wright, 80–93.

Jaspers, K. ([1913] 1997) *General Psychopathology*. Baltimore: Johns Hopkins University Press.

Kant, I. (1929) *Critique of Pure Reason*, transl. by Kemp Smith, N. London: Macmillan.

Kendell, R.E. (1975a) The concept of disease and its implications for psychiatry. *British Journal of Psychiatry* 127: 305–15.

Kendell, R.E. (1975b) *The Role of Diagnosis in Psychiatry*. Oxford: Blackwell.

Kendell, R. E. and Jablensky, A. (2003) Distinguishing between the validity and utility of psychiatric diagnoses. *American Journal of Psychiatry* 160: 4–12.

Kerlinger, F.N. (1973) *Foundations of Behavioural Research*. London: Holt, Rinehart & Winston.

Kottow, M. (2004) The battering of informed consent. *Journal of Medical Ethics* 30: 565–9.

Kripke, S. (1980) *Naming and Necessity*. Oxford: Blackwell.

Kripke, S. (1982) *Wittgenstein on Rules and Private Language*. Oxford: Blackwell.

Kupfer, D.J., First, M.B. and Regier, D.A. (Eds) (2002) *A Research Agenda for DSM–V*. Washington, DC: American Psychiatric Association.

Loewer, B. and Rey, G. (1991) *Meaning in Mind: Fodor and his critics*. Oxford: Blackwell.

Mackie, J.L. (1977) *Ethics: inventing right and wrong*. Harmondsworth: Penguin.

Mackie, J.L. (1993) Causes and conditionals. In: Sosa, E. and Tooley, M. (Eds) *Causation*. Oxford: Oxford University Press, 33–50.

Macklin, R. (2003) Applying the four principles. *Journal of Medical Ethics* 29: 275–80.

Maher, B.A. (1999) Anomalous experience in everyday life: its significance for psychopathology. *Monist* 82: 547–70.

Maier, T. (2006) Evidence-based psychiatry: understanding the limitations of a method. *Journal of Evaluation in Clinical Practice* 12: 325–9.

McDowell, J. (1998a) *Meaning, Knowledge and Reality*. Cambridge: Harvard University Press.

McDowell, J. (1998b) *Mind, Value and Reality*. Cambridge: Harvard University Press.

McMullin, E. (1987) Explanatory success and the truth of theory. In: Rescher, N. (Ed.) *Scientific Inquiry in Philosophical Perspective*. Pittsburgh: University of Pittsburgh Press, 51–73.

Megone, C. (2000) Mental illness, human function, and values. *Philosophy, Psychiatry and Psychology* 7: 45–65.

Mellor, C.S. (1970) First rank symptoms of schizophrenia. I. The frequency in schizophrenics on admission to hospital. II. Differences between individual first rank symptoms. *British Journal of Psychiatry*, 117: 15–23.

Mezzich, J.E. (2005) Values and comprehensive diagnosis. *World Psychiatry* 4: 91–2.

Mill, J.S. (1970) *A System of Logic Ratiocinative and Inductive: being a connected view of the principles of evidence and the methods of scientific investigation*. London: Longman.

Mill, J.S. (1979) *Utilitarianism*. Indianapolis: Hackett.

Millikan, R.G. (1984) *Language, Thought and other Biological Categories*. Cambridge: MIT Press.

Millikan, R.G. (1993) *White Queen Psychology*. Cambridge: MIT Press.

Millikan, R.G. (1995) A bet with Peacocke. In: Macdonald, C. and Macdonald, G. (Eds) *Philosophy of Psychology*. Oxford: Blackwell, 285–92.

Millon, T., Blaney P.H. and Davis, R.D. (1999) *Oxford Textbook of Psychopathology*. Oxford: Oxford University Press.

Mulhall, S. (1990) *On Being in the World*. London: Routledge.

Nagel, T. (1986) *The View from Nowhere*. Oxford: Oxford University Press.

Noë, A. (2004) *Action in Perception*. Cambridge: MIT Press.

Papineau, D. (1987) *Reality and Representation*. Oxford: Blackwell.

Parkin, A.J. (1996) *Explorations in Cognitive Neuropsychology*. Oxford: Blackwell.

Phillips, J. (2005) Idiographic formulations, symbols, narratives, context and meaning. *Psychopathology* 38: 180–4.

Pickering, N. (2006) *The Metaphor of Mental Illness.* Oxford: Oxford University Press.

Popper, K. (1959) *The Logic of Scientific Discovery.* New York: Basic Books.

Putnam, H. (2002) *The Collapse of the Fact/Value Dichotomy and Other Essays.* Cambridge: Harvard University Press.

Quine W.V.O. (1960) *Word and Object.* Cambridge: MIT Press.

Quine W.V.O. (1961) Two dogmas of empiricism. In: *From a Logical Point of View.* Cambridge: Harvard University Press.

Quine W.V.O. (1975) On empirically equivalent systems of the world. *Erkenntnis* 9: 313–28.

Radden, J. and Fordyce, J.M. (2006) Into the darkness: losing identity with dementia. In: Hughes *et al.* (Eds) *Dementia: mind, meaning and the person.* Oxford: Oxford University Press, 71–88.

Ramsey, F. (1931) General propositions and causality. In: Braithwaite, R.B. (Ed.) *F P Ramsey: the foundations of mathematics.* London: Routledge, 237–55.

Read, R. (2001) On approaching schizophrenia through Wittgenstein. *Philosophical Psychology* 14: 449–75.

Roessler, J. (2001) Understanding delusions of alien control. *Philosophy, Psychiatry and Psychology* 8: 177–88.

Rust, J. and Golombok, S. (1989) *Modern Psychometrics.* London: Routledge.

Ryle, G. (1949) *The Concept of Mind.* London: Hutchinson.

Sabat, S.R. (2001) *The Experience of Alzheimer's Disease.* Oxford: Blackwell.

Sabat, S.R. and Harre, R. (1994) The Alzheimer's Disease sufferer as a semiotic subject. *Philosophy, Psychiatry and Psychology* 1: 145–60.

Sackett, D.L., Straus, S.E., Richardson, W.S., Rosenberg, W. and Haynes, R.B. (2000) *Evidence-Based Medicine: how to practice and teach EBM.* Edinburgh: Churchill Livingstone.

Sadler, J.Z. (2004) *Values and Psychiatric Diagnosis.* Oxford: Oxford University Press.

Sass, L.A. (1994) *The Paradoxes of Delusion.* New York: Cornell.

Schneider, K. (1959) *Clinical Psychopathology.* New York: Grune and Stratton.

Searle, J. (1967) How to derive 'ought' from 'is'. In: Foot, P. (Ed.) *Theories of Ethics.* Oxford: Oxford University Press, 101–14.

Sellars, W. (1997) *Empiricism and the Philosophy of Mind.* Cambridge: Harvard University Press.

Shorter, E. (1997) *A History of Psychiatry.* New York: John Wiley and Sons.

Sims, A. (1988) *Symptoms in the Mind: an introduction to descriptive psychopathology.* London: Baillière Tindall.

Smith, B. (2002) Analogy in moral deliberation: the role of imagination and theory in ethics. *Journal of Medical Ethics* 28.

Smith, B. (2003) *Being in the Space of Moral Reasons: in principle and in particular,* PhD thesis submitted to the University of Warwick.

Sober, E. (1984) *The Nature of Selection.* Cambridge: MIT Press.

Spence, S.A. (1996) Free will in the light of neuropsychiatry. *Philosophy, Psychiatry and Psychology* 3: 75–90.

Stanghellini, G. (2004) *Disembodied Spirits and Deanimated Bodies.* Oxford: Oxford University Press.

Stephens, L. and Graham, G. (1994) Self-consciousness, mental agency and the clinical pathology of thought insertion. *Philosophy, Psychiatry, and Psychology* 1: 1–10.

Szasz, T. (1972) *The Myth of Mental Illness*. London: Paladin.

Szasz, T. (2004) Reply to Bentall. In: Schaler, J.A. (Ed.) *Szasz Under Fire*. Chicago: Open Court, 321–6.

Thornton, T. (1998) *Wittgenstein on Language and Thought*. Edinburgh: Edinburgh University Press.

Thornton, T. (2004) *John McDowell*. Chesham: Acumen.

Van Fraassen, B. (1980) *The Scientific Image*. Oxford: Oxford University Press.

Van Fraassen, B. (1999) To save the phenomena. In: Boyd, R., Gasker, P. and Trout, J.D. (Eds) *The Philosophy of Science*. Cambridge: MIT Press, 187–94.

Wakefield, J.C. (1992) The concept of mental disorder: on the boundary between biological facts and social values. *American Psychologist* 47: 373–88.

Wakefield, J.C. (1999) Mental disorder as a black box essentialist concept. *Journal of Abnormal Psychology* 108: 465–72.

Welsby P.D. (1999) Reductionism in medicine: some thoughts on medical education from the clinical front line. *Journal of Evaluation in Clinical Practice* 5(2): 125–31.

Whewell, W. (1849) *Of Induction, with Especial Reference to Mr. J. Stuart Mill's System of Logic*. London: Parker.

Williams D.D.R. and Garner J. (2002) The case against 'the evidence': a different perspective on evidence-based medicine. *British Journal of Psychiatry* 180, 8–12.

Winch, P. (1970) Understanding a primitive society. In: Wilson, F. (Ed.) *Rationality*. Oxford: Blackwell.

Windelband, W. ([1894] 1998) History and natural science. *Theory and Psychology* 8: 5–22.

Wittgenstein, L. (1922) *Tractatus Logico-Philosophicus*. London: Routledge.

Wittgenstein, L. (1953) *Philosophical Investigations*. Oxford: Blackwell.

Wittgenstein, L. (1969) *On Certainty*. Oxford: Blackwell.

Wittgenstein, L. (1980) *Remarks on the Philosophy of Psychology*. Oxford: Blackwell.

Wittgenstein, L. (1984) *Notebooks 1914–16*. Oxford: Blackwell.

Woodbridge, K. and Fulford, K.W.M. (2004) *Whose Values? A Workbook for Values-based Practice in Mental Health Care*. London: Sainsbury Centre for Mental Health.

Wright, C. (1986) Rule following, meaning and constructivism. In: Travis, C. (Ed.) *Meaning and Interpretation*. Oxford: Blackwell, 271–97.

Wright, C. (1987) On making up one's mind: Wittgenstein on intention. In: Weingartner, P. and Schurz, G. (Eds) *Logic, Philosophy of Science and Epistemology: Proceedings of the 11th International Wittgenstein Symposium*. Vienna: Holder-Pichler-Tempsky, 391–404.

Wright, C. (1991) Wittgenstein's later philosophy of mind: sensation, privacy and intention. In: Puhl, K. (Ed.) *Meaning Scepticism*. Berlin: de Gruyter, 126–47.

Wright, C. (1992) *Truth and Objectivity*. Cambridge: Harvard University Press.

# Guide to further reading

There is a growing literature in the philosophy of psychiatry. The journal *Philosophy, Psychiatry and Psychology* edited by Bill Fulford in the UK and John Sadler in the USA, and published by Johns Hopkins University Press, publishes original peer-reviewed articles with commentaries by philosophers and psychiatrists.

The Oxford University Press book series *International Perspectives in Philosophy and Psychiatry* edited by Bill Fulford, Katherine Morris, John Sadler and Giovanni Stanghellini already contains a number of useful works. Books in the series written by Bolton and Hill, Pickering, Sadler and Stanghellini have already been discussed in this text and others are listed in recommendations for particular chapter areas below.

In addition, however, Fulford *et al.* contains both substantial further reading itself, as well as lengthy lists for further research and Radden contains commissioned chapters on a variety of topics:

Fulford, K.W.M., Thornton, T. and Graham, G. (2006) *Oxford Textbook of Philosophy and Psychiatry*. Oxford: Oxford University Press.

Radden, J. (Ed.) (2004) *The Philosophy of Psychiatry: a companion*. New York: Oxford University Press.

The series launch volume has both a variety of original papers drawing on both continental and analytic philosophy, and a useful introduction to the subject area.

Fulford, K.W.M, Morris, K., Sadler, J. and Stanghellini, G. (Eds) (2003) *Nature and Narrative*. Oxford: Oxford University Press.

In addition to the Oxford University Press *International Perspectives in Philosophy and Psychiatry* series, there is also Gerrit Glas' series in Dutch, the *Psychiatry and Philosophy* book series from Boom Publishers in Amsterdam, a series from Martin Heinze's group in Germany, the GPWP (Gesellschaft für Philosophie und Wissenschaften der Psyche), and from France a new review published by PSN-Edition in Paris, *Psychiatrie, Sciences Humaines et Neurosciences*.

## Part I: Values

### 1. Anti-psychiatry, values and the philosophy of psychiatry

In addition to Szasz' work, the other main sources for anti-psychiatric argument are, from a phenomenological perspective Laing (1960) and from a historical, albeit philosophically-informed, perspective Foucault (1965):

Laing, R.D. (1960) *The Divided Self*. London: Tavistock Publications.
Foucault, M. (1965) *Madness and Civilisation*. New York: Mentor Books.

A recent edited collection on Laing is:

Rascid, S. (Ed.) (2005) *RD Laing Contemporary Perspectives*, London: Free Association Books.

A good critique of Foucault is:

Matthews, E. (1995) Moralist or therapist? Foucault and the critique of psychiatry. *Philosophy, Psychiatry and Psychology* 2: 19–30.

Many of the most important classic papers in the debate about mental illness are gathered in:

Caplan, A.L., Engelhardt, H.J. and McCartney, J.J. (Eds) (1981) *Concepts of Health and Disease*. Reading: Addison-Wesley Publishing.

More recent reviews include an entry on 'Mental Illness' by Fulford, K.W.M., cited in:

Chadwick, R. (Ed) (1998) *The Encyclopedia of Applied Ethics*. San Diego: Academic Press.
Gert, B. and Culver, C.M. (2004) Defining mental disorder. In: Radden, J (Ed.) *The Philosophy of Psychiatry: a companion*. Oxford: Oxford University Press.

A distinct theory of the connection between illness and values is articulated by Lennart Nordenfelt in:

Nordenfelt, L. (1987) *On the Nature of Health: an action-theoretic account of health*. Dordrecht: D. Redel Publishing.
Nordenfelt, L. (1997) *Talking about Health: a philosophical dialogue*. Amsterdam: Rodopi.
Nordenfelt, L. (2001) *Health, Science and Ordinary Language*. Amsterdam: Rodopi.

For a perspective on the debate that draws on ancient philosophy, see:

Matthews, E. (1999) Moral vision and the idea of mental illness. *Philosophy, Psychiatry and Psychology* 6: 299–310.

In 2000, *Philosophy, Psychiatry and Psychology* published a special edition comparing the idea that mental disorder is genuinely teleological with the idea that it is a failure of biological function. This included critical articles by both Szasz and Wakefield and a substantial reply by:

Megone, C. (2000) Mental illness, human function, and values. *Philosophy, Psychiatry and Psychology* 7: 45–65.

A more general collection on the philosophy of biological functions is:

Allen, C. and Lauder, G. (Eds) *Nature's Purposes: analyses of function and design in biology.* Cambridge: MIT Press.

In 2005, *Philosophy, Psychiatry and Psychology* published a special issue on Mild Cognitive Impairment with an introduction by:

Hughes, J.C. (2005) Introduction: the heat of mild cognitive impairment. *Philosophy, Psychiatry and Psychology* 13: 1–2.

## 2. Values, psychiatric ethics and clinical judgement

There is a very large introductory literature on moral philosophy and ethics generally, but one book that explicitly contrasts Kantian, consequentialist and virtue ethical approaches is by:

Baron, M.W., Petit, P. and Slote, M. (1997) *Three Methods of Ethics: a debate.* Oxford: Blackwell.

Bioethics is similarly large and a growing field, but one general book of particular relevance to the philosophy of psychiatry is:

Gillett, G.R. (2004) *Bioethics in the Clinic.* Baltimore: Johns Hopkins University Press.

There are two related collections on psychiatric ethics, together with a related workbook by:

Bloch, S., Chodoff, P. and Green, S.A. (Eds) *Psychiatric Ethics*, 3rd edn. Oxford: Oxford University Press.

Dickenson, D. and Fulford, K.W.M. (Eds) *In Two Minds: a casebook of psychiatric ethics.* Oxford: Oxford University Press.

Green, S. and Bloch, S. (Eds) *An Anthology of Psychiatric Ethics.* Oxford: Oxford University Press.

For an account of the relation between the use of mental illness as a defence, and moral and legal assumptions see:

Robinson, D.N. (2000) Madness, badness, and fitness: law and psychiatry (again). *Philosophy, Psychiatry and Psychology* 7: 209–22.

Particularist approaches to moral philosophy are defended by Jonathan Dancy:

Dancy, J. (1993) *Moral Reasons*. Oxford: Blackwell.

Dancy, J. (2006) *Ethics Without Principles*. Oxford: Oxford University Press.

The broader account of nature into which this fits is set out in:

Dancy, J. (2000) *Practical reality*. Oxford: Oxford University Press.

A good introduction to the arguments for and against moral particularism is:

McNaughton, D. (1998) *Moral vision*. Oxford: Blackwell.

In 2003, the *Journal of Medical Ethics* published a festschrift edition in honour of Raanan Gillon, containing a number of papers examining the Four Principles approach to medical ethics and with an editorial of interest:

Savulescu, J. (2003) Editorial: promoting respect for the four principles remains of great practical importance in ordinary medicine. *Journal of Medical Ethics*, 29: 265–6.

## Part II: Meanings

### 3. Understanding psychopathology

The following set out both introductions to Jaspers and to his influence on psychiatry:

Hoenig, J. (1965) Karl Jaspers and psychopathology. *Philosophy and Phenomenological Research* 26: 216–29.

Schlipp, P.A. (1981) *The Philosophy of Karl Jaspers*. LaSalle: Open Court.

Shepherd, M. (1990) *Karl Jaspers: general psychopathology, Conceptual Issues in Psychological Medicine*. London: Tavistock.

Schmitt, W. (1986) Karl Jaspers' influence on psychiatry. *Journal of the British Society for Phenomenology* 17: 36–51.

A critical view of Jaspers' phenomenology is given in:

Bracken, P. and Thomas, P. (2005) *Postpsychiatry*. Oxford: Oxford University Press.

Theory theory and simulation theory have recently been discussed as rival theories in a number of collections of papers:

Davies, M. and Stone, T. (Eds) (1995) *Folk Psychology: a guide to the theory of mind debate*. Oxford: Blackwell.

Davies, M. and Stone, T. (Eds) (1995) *Mental Simulation: evaluations and applications*. Oxford: Blackwell.

Carruthers, P. and Smith, P.K. (Eds) (1996) *Theories of Theories of Mind*. Cambridge: Cambridge University Press.

Psychotic experiences have received particular attention in *Philosophy, Psychiatry and Psychology*. The first article in the first issue was on thought insertion:

Stephens, G.L. and Graham, G. (1994) Self-consciousness, mental agency and the clinical psychopathology of thought insertion. *Philosophy, Psychiatry and Psychology* 1: 1–10.

In 2001 there was a special edition edited, and with an introduction, by Christoph Hoerl:

Hoerl, C. (2001) Introduction: understanding, explaining and intersubjectivity in schizophrenia. *Philosophy, Psychiatry and Psychology* 8: 83–88.

This edition also contains articles by both analytic and continental philosophers.

In addition, there are a number of edited collections in book form. These include:

Chung, M.C., Fulford, K.W.M. and Graham, G. (Eds) (2006) *Reconceiving Schizophrenia*. Oxford: Oxford University Press

Coltheart, M and Davies, M. (Eds) (2000) *Pathologies of Delusion*. Oxford: Blackwell

Graham, G. and Stephens, G.L. (Eds) (1995) *Philosophical Psychopathology*. Cambridge: MIT Press

Graham, G. and Stephens, G.L. (Eds) (2000) *When Self-Consciousness Breaks: Alien voices and inserted thoughts*. Cambridge: MIT Press.

By contrast with psychotic experience, a useful collection on the philosophical understanding of dementia is:

Hughes, J., Louw, S. and Sabat, S. (Eds) (2005) *Dementia: mind, meaning and the person*. Oxford: Oxford University Press.

## 4. Theorising about meaning for mental health care

Useful introductions to the philosophy of content or intentionality can be found in the general philosophy of mind textbook:

Braddon-Mitchell, D. and Jackson, F. (1996) *Philosophy of Mind and Cognition*. Oxford: Blackwell, chapters 10–11.

They can also be found in textbooks on the philosophy of content specifically. See, for example:

Luntley, M.O. (1999) *Contemporary Philosophy of Thought*. Oxford: Blackwell.

Miller, A. (1998) *The Philosophy of Language*. London: UCL.
Representationalism is defended in:

Sterelny, K. (1990) *The Representational Theory of Mind*. Oxford: Blackwell.

The language of thought is discussed in the appendix to:

Fodor, J. (1987) *Psychosemantics*. Cambridge: MIT Press.

Ruth Millikan's work is set out fully in:

Millikan, R. (1984) *Language Thought and other Biological Categories*. Cambridge: MIT Press.

Millikan, R. (1993) *White Queen Psychology*. Cambridge: MIT Press.

Concise introductions are:

Macdonald, G. (1995) The biological turn. In: Macdonald, C. and Macdonald, G. (Eds) *Philosophy of Psychology*. Oxford: Blackwell, 238–51.

Millikan, R. (1995) Biosemantics: explanation in biopsychology. In: Macdonald, C. and Macdonald, G. (Eds) *Philosophy of Psychology*. Oxford: Blackwell, 252–76.

Clinical work in a cognitive neuropsychological framework can be found in:

Caramazza, A. (Ed.) (1999) *Cognitive Neuropsychology and Neurolinguistics*. Baltimore: Johns Hopkins University Press.

For a Wittgensteinian critique of representationalism see:

Thornton, T. (1998) *Wittgenstein on Language and Thought*. Edinburgh: Edinburgh University Press.

Interesting interdisciplinary work can be found in:

Carruthers, P. and Boucher, J. (Eds) *Language and Thought: interdisciplinary themes*. Cambridge: Cambridge University Press.

The discursive approach to psychology is outlined in a number of places:

Church, J. (2004) Social constructionist models: making order out of disorder—on the social construction of madness. In: Radden, J. (Ed.) *The Philosophy of Psychiatry*. Oxford: Oxford University Press.

Edwards, D. and Potter, J. (1992) *Discursive Psychology*. London: Sage.

Harré, R. and Gillett, G. (1994) *The Discursive Mind*. London: Sage.

There is a very great deal written on the interpretation of Wittgenstein's *Philosophical Investigations* (1953). A good place to start, with critical discussion of Kripke, Wright and McDowell is:

McGinn, M. (1999) *Wittgenstein's Philosophical Investigations*. London: Routledge.

Thornton, T. (1998) *Wittgenstein on Language and Thought*. Edinburgh: Edinburgh University Press.

A good collection of essays on Wittgenstein's discussion of rules can be found in:

Miller, A. and Wright, C. (Eds) (2002) *Rule-Following and Meaning*. Chesham: Acumen.

A useful beginning to Dennett's philosophy of mind is his:

Dennett, D.C. (1996) *Kinds of Minds*. New York: Basic Books.

A clear statement of Davidson's philosophy is:

Davidson, D. (1984) Belief and the basis of meaning. In: Davidson, D. (Ed.) *Inquiries into Truth and Interpretation*. Oxford: Oxford University Press, 141–54.

Davidson's philosophy is introduced in:

Evnine, S. (1991) *Donald Davidson*. Oxford: Polity.

# Part III: Facts

## 5. The validity of psychiatric classification

Two useful, contrasting introductions to the philosophy of science as a whole are:

Bird, A. (1998) *The Philosophy of Science*. London: Routledge

Chalmers, A.F. (1999) *What is this Thing called Science?* Indianapolis: Hackett Publishing Company.

A substantial collection of philosophy of science papers is:

Boyd, R., Gasker, P. and Trout, J.D. (Eds) (1999) *The Philosophy of Science*. Cambridge: MIT Press.

The definitive collection on scientific realism is:

Leplin, J. (Ed.) (1984) *Scientific Realism*. Berkeley: University of California. It is also discussed in:

Papineau, D. (1987) *Reality and Representation*. Oxford: Blackwell.

Laudan, L. (1977) *Progress and its Problems*. Berkeley: University of California.

Scientific realism based on the argument from explanation is the main subject of:

Lipton, P. (1999) *Inference to the Best Explanation*. London: Routledge.

One debate that has not been touched on in this chapter concerns whether disease is a natural kind. See, for example:

Reznek, L. (1987) *The Nature of Disease*. London: Routledge.

Reznek, L. (1995) Dis-ease about kinds: reply to D'Amico. *Journal of Medicine and Philosophy* 20: 571–84.

D'Amico, R. (1995) Is disease a natural kind? *Journal of Medicine and Philosophy* 20: 551–69.

Key philosophical discussions of psychiatric taxonomy include:

Cooper, R. (2005) *Classifying Madness: a philosophical examination of the Diagnostic and Statistical Manual of Mental Disorders*. Dordrecht: Springer.

Sadler, J.Z., Wiggins, O.P. and Schwartz, M.A. (Eds) (1994) *Philosophical Perspectives on Psychiatric Diagnostic Classification*. Baltimore: Johns Hopkins University Press.

The role of values within scientific psychiatry and especially classification is thoroughly investigated in:

Sadler, J.Z. (2004) *Values and Psychiatric Diagnosis*. Oxford: Oxford University Press.

For a critique of the criteriological model of diagnosis from a phenomenological perspective see:

Kraus, A. (1994) Phenomenological and criteriological diagnosis. In: Sadler, J.Z., Wiggins, O.P. and Schwartz, M.A. (Eds) *Philosophical Perspectives on Psychiatric Diagnostic Classification*. Baltimore: Johns Hopkins University Press.

## 6. The relation of evidence-based medicine and tacit knowledge in clinical judgement

A thorough practical introduction to EBM is provided by:

Sackett, D.L., Straus, S.E., Richardson, W.S., Rosenberg, W. and Haynes, R.B. (2000) *Evidence-based Medicine: how to practice and teach EBM*. Edinburgh: Churchill Livingstone.

Hume's philosophy is described in a number of introductions including:

Pears, D. (1990) *Hume's System*. Oxford: Oxford University Press
Stroud, B. (1977) *Hume*. London: Routledge.

The problem of induction is thoroughly set out and a particular solution suggested in:

Howson, C. (2000) *Hume's Problem: induction and the justification of belief*. Oxford: Clarendon.

The clearest short account of how Mill's methods work is contained within:

Copi, I.M. (1984) *Introduction to Logic*. London: Macmillan.

This also provides a thorough introduction to logical reasoning.
Popper's falsificationism is introduced in:

Bird, A. (1998) *The Philosophy of Science*. London: Routledge.
Chalmers, A.F. (1999) *What is this Thing called Science?* Indianapolis: Hackett Publishing Company.
Popper, K. (1959) *The Logic of Scientific Discovery*. New York: Basic Books.

The method of clinical trials is set out in:

Pocock, S.J. (1983) *Clinical Trials: a practical approach*. New York: John Wiley and Sons Ltd.

Although not described in this chapter, the connection between the analysis of causal connections and necessity and sufficiency was influentially examined in:

Mackie, J.L. (1993) Causes and conditionals. In: Sosa, E. and Tooley, M. (Eds) *Causation*. Oxford: Oxford University Press, 33–50.

The use of causation in medical diagnosis is described in the articles:

Rizzi, D.A. (1994) Causal reasoning and the diagnostic process. *Theoretical Medicine* 15: 315–33.

Lindahl, I.B. and Nordenfelt, L. (Eds) (1984) *Health, Disease, and Causal Explanations in Medicine*. Dordrecht: Reidel Publishing Company.

Books that claim an important role for tacit knowledge in science include:

Collins, H. (1985) *Changing Order: replication and induction in scientific practice*. London: Sage.

Kuhn, T. (1962) *The Structure of Scientific Revolutions*. Chicago: University of Chicago Press.

Polanyi, M. (1967) *The Tacit Dimension*. London: Routledge.

A criticism of an overemphasis on science in psychiatry is put forward in:

Bracken, P. and Thomas, P. (2005) *Postpsychiatry*. Oxford: Oxford University Press.

# Sources

Whilst I have aimed in this book to present a coherent overview of the philosophy of psychiatry that reflects the state of play across the three areas of values, meanings and facts, I have borrowed and reworked some material that I have published elsewhere into different chapters here. I would like to thank the publishers for permission to do this.

## 1. Anti-psychiatry, values and the philosophy of psychiatry

Thornton, T. (2000) Mental illness and reductionism: can functions be naturalized? *Philosophy, Psychiatry and Psychology* 7: 67–76.

Thornton, T. (2004) Reductionism/anti-reductionism, in J. Radden (Ed.) *The Philosophy of Psychiatry*. Oxford: Oxford University Press, 191–204.

Thornton, T. (2006) The ambiguities of mild cognitive impairment. *Philosophy, Psychiatry and Psychology* 13: 21–27.

## 2. Values, psychiatric ethics and clinical judgement

Thornton, T. (2004) *John McDowell*. Chesham: Acumen, chapter 2.

Thornton, T. (2006) Judgement and the role of the metaphysics of values in medical ethics. *Journal of Medical Ethics* 32: 365–370.

## 3. Understanding psychopathology

Thornton, T. (2004) Wittgenstein and the limits of empathic understanding in psychopathology. *International Review of Psychiatry* 16: 216–224.

## 4. Theorising about meaning for mental health care

Thornton, T. (2002) Thought insertion, cognitivism and inner space. *Cognitive Neuropsychiatry* 7: 237–249.

Thornton, T. (2005) Discursive psychology, social constructionism and dementia, in J. Hughes, S. Louw and S. Sabat (Eds) *Dementia: mind, meaning and the person*. Oxford: Oxford University Press 123–141.

## 5. The validity of psychiatric classification

Thornton, T. (2002) Reliability and validity in psychiatric classification: values and *neo-Humanism*. *Philosophy, Psychiatry and Psychology* 9: 229–235.

Thornton, T. (2006) In: Fulford, K.W.M, Thornton, T. and Graham, G. (Eds) *The Oxford Textbook of Philosophy and Psychiatry*. Oxford: Oxford University Press, chapter 13.

## 6. The relation of evidence-based medicine and tacit knowledge in clinical judgement

Thornton, T. (2006) In: Fulford, K.W.M, Thornton, T. and Graham, G. (Eds) *The Oxford Textbook of Philosophy and Psychiatry*. Oxford: Oxford University Press, chapter 16.

# Index

*Note to index:* for definitions and explanations refer to the *glossary of philosophical terms* on pp. 239–43